CHICKEN SOUP
For Your FUTURE

PHIL SUMNER

Order this book online at www.trafford.com
or email orders@trafford.com

Most Trafford titles are also available at major online book retailers.

Printed in the United States of America.

ISBN: 978-1-4669-5335-2 (sc)

Trafford rev. 11/07/2012

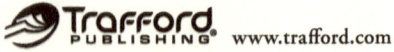 www.trafford.com

North America & international
toll-free: 1 888 232 4444 (USA & Canada)
phone: 250 383 6864 ♦ fax: 812 355 4082

Contents

Introduction

HOW WOULD YOU like to add an extra 10 years to your life??? An enjoyable 10 years? It is now possible with health and life approaches discussed in this book. And if 10 years is acceptable to you, how about 15 years? 20 years? Or 50 years?

I am personally looking forward to my next 20 years. And at the end of that 20 years, I now plan to enjoy another 20 years. And another 20. Would you like to join me? I am personally looking forward to what the future will bring. And this means that I have high hopes for the future. Again, care to join me?

To achieve these health benefits, you will probably need to change your life style, perhaps drastically in some cases. For example, if you smoke, then quit. Right now.

The human race is in for some radical changes in the next 50 years, and most of them will be good for us; we will look back then and like what we see. We are in for a literal explosion in human abilities. We will be smarter, be healthier, live longer, be very much kinder to our neighbors, and be much more aware of our surroundings and its limitless possibilities. And I see this coming due to the cumulative effects of several major characteristics that are evident now, but which have not been explored in this context.

This book is my honest look at what your future might hold. I discuss the medical and life changing impacts on your future. There will be some things familiar to you, and probably some new things. It just might give you a new direction, a new approach, or a different way of looking at things, and hopefully resulting in a better, longer, and more healthful life. I therefore wish you a mostly disease-free, longer, and more healthful life.

This book is applicable to all ages. The elder generation can use this advice to retrieve what health they should have had and live the rest of their life, possibly many years longer than they would have otherwise. The middle generation can use it to eliminate many illnesses that otherwise would have incapacitated them, thus allowing them to live joyfully much longer. The current younger generation can use this to avoid illnesses along the way to growing old, and therefore will live longer. I believe that this group can expect to live past 100, and thoroughly enjoy that life past 90. And those still to be born will grow up with habits and nutrition that will naturally let them live past 100, with many of them going to 120 and beyond. I have seen one report that projects the human life span to 150 by 2050. Read on! Enjoy!

Abnormally Normal

Looking back at my life, I have recently thought,
That it seems I've been caught in a web I've not wrought.
Some unfriendly old fiend has been running the show—
I could only stop short, when I wanted to go;
Or the inverse of this, like some idiot swap,
I could only keep mov'n when I wanted to stop.

After a week of hard work, with much more as the trend,
I was primed for relaxing and fun at the end;
Friday night all these plans were upset rather much—
My wife hinted at painting, yard work and such.

For my favorite program I'd waited all week,
But at my favorite last Friday, there wasn't a peek;
The announcement was made with a voice so genial—
"Ladies and Gentlemen, the Friday Special!"

Disenchanted with streets, with their drivers so deft,
With their circles and signals and cars turning left,
I thought maybe the freeway was the home route that's fast—
But the traffic on that road just left me aghast!

I came home from work tired, just wanting to sit
With a good ice-cold beer and relax for a bit;
Disillusionment, though, settled in mighty swift—
Oh, Lord! It's her birthday—I don't have a gift!

Phil Sumner

For two weeks I had dreaded that monthly due date—
At long last, I resigned to my miserable fate.
The bills had to be paid—I began that sad chore—
Then a so-called good friend sauntered in from next door.

In the hectic preparation for dinner for eight,
The neighborhood gossip dropped in and stayed late,
Until I was convinced it had gone much too far,
And that friend should be spelled by omitting the R.

There are times when I wonder at odd things like these,
Whether I've been afflicted by Job's non-disease.
But if others could analyze, probe, and then judge
My life as it has been, the grandeur and sludge,
Then report it, I think their conclusion I'd know—
That I seem more than ever like Tom, Dick, and Joe.

Chapter 1
Medical Supplements

WOULDN'T IT BE wonderful to have good health all the time? To not worry about colds or flu or any other diseases that might be going around? To know that, short of some fatal disease or accident, we had the expectation of living past 90? Or 105 (in a very few years)? Or 150 (by 2050)?

There are many things you can do for yourself to enhance your health and therefore your enjoyment of life, and also extend the enjoyable portion of your life. The more you can assume of the responsibilities for your future, the better off you will be. And isn't a longer, more healthy, and more enjoyable life worth setting as a major goal?

One way you probably need to change your life style is that you need to take medical supplements, defined as non-prescription medication. You cannot get everything you need for a nominal, healthy life from diet alone, and prescriptions are given to "fix" existing problems. Which means you need to become a "pill popper" if you are not already. And if you presently cannot take pills, then learn how; practice makes perfect. To be healthy, happy, and "with it" in life, pills are in your future; all the supplements needed cannot be obtained in liquid form.

My present recommendations for medical supplements are given below. Please note that these are mostly arranged in the order of importance; the most important supplements are always listed as **major** somewhere in the presentation. I also try to give a source for each recommendation, along with a nominal "cost" of each "bottle" or other container and the daily cost of each supplement; this may help you to make an intelligent decision as to which ones to try. If your funds are unlimited, feel free to enjoy all of them; I use them myself, and vouch for them. But if your funds are limited, look at the top supplements and go for them first.

Please note that you will not necessarily notice any improvements or any changes at all when taking these supplements. But if you follow my recommendations, then I strongly believe that you will wake up 5 or 10 years down the road feeling better, enjoying life more, and liking how you feel and live. Read on! Enjoy!

In many places in this book, I give the name, address, and phone number of many companies "out there". These are listed simply because I personally have knowledge of them. But be aware that there are many companies that are not in business to help you, but instead want to make a quick buck. Products from these companies are likely to be bogus, and might even be dangerous. Please use common sense when dealing with these other companies.

Centrum Silver Multivitamin (Seniors older than about 60)

Use: General health; everyone needs a good multivitamin each day. It is a particularly good source of many trace minerals that your body needs but comes from no other source.

Source: Wal-Mart

Cost: $7.20 for 100, or 7 cents per day, Wal-Mart

Any good multivitamin (Everyone else)

Use: General health; everyone needs a good multivitamin each day. It is a particularly good source of many trace minerals that your body needs but comes from no other source.

Source: Any good drug store or via the Internet

Cost: unknown, but anything less than $10 per hundred would be reasonable.

Fish Oil, 1 to 3 g, Everyone

Use: Used for general health throughout your body. The Omega 3 oil has multiple benefits, such as: increases the levels of "good" cholesterol in your bloodstream, improves your cardiovascular system, improves heart and eye health, improves memory and brain function, reduces allergies, strengthens your bones, makes your skin more radiant, and supports a healthy inflammation response. Fish oil is a **MAJOR** benefit to the body.

Source: Wal-Mart for the garden variety of fish oil (better than nothing and relatively inexpensive), or Life Extension Foundation for an advanced version of fish oil that has less contaminants and can be taken in higher dosages without repercussions like bloating, contaminants, or gas. The higher you go in quantity, the more contaminants become an issue in taking Fish Oil. If this is an issue with you, please see the pharmaceutical grade fish oil and the Krill Oil options discussed below.

Cost: $11.94 for 250 softgels or 125 days, about 9.5 cents a day from Wal-Mart. Another option for this is called "One Per Day" Omega 3 Fish Oil, and it has double the usual content; I found this at Wal-Mart recently. So only 1 capsule needs to be taken per day. The cost of this option is $9.76 for 90 softgels, or a little less than 11 cents a day. The version of fish oil that comes from Life Extension Foundation is called Super Omega-3; the 120 softgels in each bottle costs $32.00 for a non-member, or $24.00 for a member. Alternatively, a member can purchase 4 bottles for $21.00 per bottle. At 2 softgels taken per day, this works out to a 60-day supply in each bottle, or about 35 cents per day. In my own mind, this is worth it; I have switched to it.

Another option for taking fish oil has recently come to my attention. This was via a very good book titled *The Omega RX Zone* by Dr. Barry Sears. He strongly recommends taking high dose fish oil, but only if it is pharmaceutical grade, which has the usual contaminants, removed and tastes good (not at all like your grandmother's Cod Liver Oil). The major problem with this is obtaining a source. Dr. Sears lists one source in his book, but it is undoubtedly expensive. Another source for something close to pharmaceutical grade is the fish oil from Life Extension Foundation, which is double refined and thus causes less bloating and gas.

Still another source of Omega 3 fish oils is from a small crustacean living at the bottom of the world. These little animals are called krill, and form the main diet of some whales. For our purposes, krill oil is several times more bio-available than standard fish oil, and naturally contains none of the bothersome contaminants like lead, mercury, and others that are found in normal fish oil. So krill oil can be taken in dosages high enough to assist in the most bothersome conditions, and without the burps and bad taste. If this is interesting to you, check out Health Resources, 904 Ploof Drive, Hueytown AL 35023, 1-800-471-4007. Their krill oil is called Super Krill-Omega3 and costs $339 for a 12-month supply.

Special Note: If you are in dire straits heart-wise and want to pursue pharmaceutical grade fish oil, the single source recommended in *The Omega RX Zone* is Sears Lab, 1-800-404-8171. If this is important to you, please check into it and let me know. Or check out the krill oil option discussed above.

Another special note: if you are taking the Life Extension fish oil and need something more, take as many as 6 of their soft gels daily; three in the morning, and 3 in the evening. If this causes objectionable bloating or gas, cut back to 3 soft gels. Or check out the Sears Lab discussed in the previous paragraph. Or check out the krill oil option discussed above.

CoQ10, 200 mg of the garden variety (ubiquonone), or 50 mg or more of the variety from Life Extension Foundation (Super Ubiquinol); everyone past about age 35 and interested in a longer and happier, more disease-free life.

Use: Used for general health throughout your body, in every cell in your body. Super Ubiquinol is an effective scavenger of free radicals, and is more readily available for energy production in the mitochondria, the energy workhorses in each cell. It also slows the signs of aging and is more effective at combating fatigue. It is a **MAJOR** benefit to the body. You should also be prepared for your libido to increase; in other words, your sex life might get into a higher gear.

Source: Life Extension Foundation (www.lef.org) for Super Ubiquinol CoQ10 or call them at 1-800-544-4440. I use and recommend this version. Another source of the apparently good CoQ10 is BioNutrigenics, which has a product called Ubitol (www.ubitol.com), or call them at 1-800-207-5108. I have no personal knowledge about Ubitol, but another person I know is using it and is happy. Still another source of the apparently good CoQ10 is Forward Nutrition, which has a product called BioActive Q; call them at 1-800-211-8560. I know nothing about this version and therefore cannot recommend it. Still another source of the good CoQ10 has been identified, and the pattern seems to be now set. The more bio-available form of CoQ10 is now available from many sources, but the version from Life Extension still has my vote; it is about twice as bio-available as the others, due to their "patented delivery system".

Cost: $15.36 for 30, or about 51 cents per day at Wal-Mart for the ubiquonone variety. The recommended version (Super Ubiquinol CoQ10) from Life Extension Foundation is $58.00 for 100 of the 50 mg softgels, or about 58 cents per day for non-members. If you become a member and buy 4 bottles at a time, the price reduces to $37.50 per bottle ($150.00 total order), or about 37 cents a day. The Ubitol from BioNutrigenics is $59.95 for a 30 day supply, or about 50 cents a day. The BioActive Q from Forward Nutrition is normally $26.99 for a 30-day supply of 30 mg softgels, or about 90 cents per day.

The recommended version of CoQ10 is highly absorbable and is therefore more available to all your body cells. CoQ10 is expensive, but very much worth it. As stated above, my recommendation for obtaining this essential nutrient is Life Extension Foundation.

Vitamin D3, at least 7000 IU, everyone past the age of about 20.

Use: Required to work with Calcium to protect against weak bones. Vitamin D3 also helps with 17 varieties of cancer, heart disease, stroke, hypertension, autoimmune diseases, diabetes, depression, chronic pain, osteoarthritis, osteoporosis, muscle wasting, birth defects, periodontal disease, and helps people to live longer.

Vitamin D3 is a **MAJOR** player, and you cannot get enough through diet alone or via sunshine on your skin. To determine what you need, add up the Vitamin D3 you get in your Calcium and your multivitamin, and then take as many individual Vitamin D3 pills as necessary to achieve the daily maintenance dose of 7000 to 10,000 IU.

When first increasing the dosage of Vitamin D3, take as much as 20,000 IU per day to "load" your system for a couple of months, then phase back to around 7000 to 10,000 IU as a maintenance dose. The more Vitamin D3 you take, the better it is for you. The increased dosage suggestion is due to Vitamin D3's ability to eliminate the flu virus, including Swine Flu, in addition to its other **major** benefits.

Anyone subscribing to my recommendations on Vitamin D3 should consult with their doctor or other medical provider before doing so. And they should get a test reading of their blood level of Vitamin D3 to verify that their blood level of 25-hydroxyvitamin D is at least 50 ng/ml. Once you get a blood level reading like that, you can phase back to 7,000 to 10,000 IU of Vitamin D3 per day. And if your doctor does not agree with my recommendations, and does not want to verify them, feel free to find yourself another doctor. My recommendations are based on new data that has been recently released by Life Extension, so the average doctor would be unaware of them.

Source: Wal-Mart

Cost: $6.44 for 200 tablets of 400 IU each, or just over 3 cents each day. Similar costs are available for bottles of 5000 IU and 2000 IU.

Additional data on Vitamin D3 is contained in Appendix 1.

Vitamin K, Everyone, especially those taking Vitamin D3.

Use: Vitamin K is a helper to Vitamin D3. Vitamin K plays a critical role in maintaining healthy bone density by facilitating the transport of calcium from the bloodstream into the bone. Vitamin K is also required by calcium-regulating proteins in the arteries. Vitamin K has also been proven to be an excellent "drug" against cancer; stay tuned on this one. So Vitamin K has been added to my list of **MAJOR** supplements that you should be taking.

Vitamin K comes in 3 flavors, K1, MK-4, and MK-7, and all 3 flavors are valuable in the body. However, only K1 is available from normal diet sources, but very little of that is actually absorbed; K1 is usually bound too tight to the vegetable molecules.

Source: The only source of Vitamin K that I would presently recommend is from Life Extension (http://www.lef.org/), (1-800-544-4440) for Super K with Advanced K2 Complex. This has all 3 flavors of Vitamin K in it, in about the same ratio needed by the body. I know of no other source for Vitamin K, including Wal-Mart.

Cost: $17.25 per bottle if a member buys 4 bottles. Each bottle contains 90 softgels, for a daily cost of 19 cents.

Special note: Since I have been taking Vitamin K, my world has "opened up" a little more. I feel like doing things again, feel better, sleep better, etc. All good things.

Additional data on Vitamin K is contained in Appendix 2.

Metformin. Everyone past the age of about 20.

Use: Like Vitamin K, Metformin is an excellent cancer fighter. It currently fights Breast Cancer, Endometrial Cancer, Prostate Cancer, Pancreatic Cancer, and Colon Cancer. It probably fights almost every developmental stage in almost every cancer in existence. This is currently being tested in many laboratories in the world, so stay tuned on this one.

Metformin is a prescription drug, currently the most popular diabetes drug, taken by thousands if not millions of people. The generic version of this is available and currently inexpensive, so a prescription from your doctor for this should not break the bank.

Source: Almost any drug supply house, including your neighborhood pharmacy. The generic version of Metformin is what you want, and the prescription from your doctor can be used almost anywhere. I plan to use mine with my prescription provider for a 90-day supply.

One precaution. When I took Metformin, I had an adverse reaction to it; if I remember right, I had jitters and other indications of a lower blood sugar. If Metformin works on you like it did on me, and this is objectionable, then by all means discontinue taking it. As in all things medical, talk to your doctor.

Cost: This is still to be determined, but it should be low for the generic version.

A more complete description of Metformin is contained in Appendix 3.

Vitamin C, 1000 mg, everyone
Use: Vitamin C is a general antioxidant, used throughout your body to neutralize free radicals and other duties.
Source: Wal-Mart or any other drug store
Cost: $11.26 for 250 tablets of 1000 mg each, or 125 days, just over 9 cents a day.

Ester-C, 1000 mg, everyone that cannot take the standard Vitamin C, which was my case. After taking Nexium for several years, my system was apparently switched to produce a sour stomach if I go off Nexium. A standard Vitamin C tablet is sour enough to set me off big time if I do nothing else. So this item is a choice you can make; either the standard Vitamin C or the Ester-C.

Special Note: After working with this combination for several months, I finally settled on taking the standard

Vitamin C pill, but taking it separate from my other pills; in almost all cases, the pill went down OK. This resolved my problems with a sticky throat, heartburn, and Vitamin C.

Source: Wal-Mart

Cost: $13.92 for 120 coated tablets, for 60 days, or about 23 cents a day.

Calcium, 1200 mg, everyone past about age 30

Use: Protects against weak bones, which everyone is susceptible to (even men). Buy your calcium with as much Vitamin D3 included as you can find.

Source: Wal-Mart or any other drug store

Cost: $5.97 for 250 tablets of 600 mg each, or 125 days, less than 5 cents per day.

Vitamin E, 400 IU, everyone

Use: Used as a blood thinner as protection against strokes, as an antioxidant in many places, and multiple other things in the body.

Source: Vitamin World at Rockvale Outlets near Lancaster PA, or the Internet at (http://www. vitaminworld.com/); their Vitamin E has all 4 "flavors" (alpha, beta, gamma, and delta tocopherols) of vitamin E in it, which is much better than Vitamin E from Wal-Mart or any other drug store. The standard version of Vitamin E has only alpha tocopherol in it, which is useful and needed, but gamma tocopherol also has a large benefit to the body. And please note: alpha tocopherol erodes gamma tocopherol in the body, and therefore is injurious to the body. Bottom line; take the full-flavored variety, with all 4 flavors. Check the label of any bottle you plan to buy to verify that all 4 flavors are present.

Cost: $19.99 per 250 softgels, or a little over 8 cents a day

Aspirin, 325 mg if subject to strokes, otherwise a baby aspirin of 85 mg per day, each day; everyone past about age 25

Use: Blood thinner, protects against stroke. Heart protector in many ways, but don't take other NSAIDs or the aspirin will lose its heart-healthy benefits

Source: Wal-Mart or any drug store

Cost: minimal

A more complete discussion of Aspirin is contained in Appendix 4.

Vitamin B-12, 1000 mcg, everyone over about 40 years old.

Use: Essential for cell growth and replication. It helps form red blood cells; helps maintain normal levels of homocysteine, which is important for heart and circulatory health; and plays an important role in the nervous system and proper function of all body, brain, and nerve cells. Take with Folic Acid, next.

Source: Wal-Mart

Cost: $9.28 for 250 tablets, or about 3.7 cents per day

Folic Acid, 800 mcg, everyone over about 40 years of age
Use: Overall body health; works synergistically with Vitamin B-12. In addition, it is an excellent scavenger of free radicals, helps protect chromosomes against genetic damage, helps prevent pregnancy defects, participates in the utilization of sugar and carbohydrates, promotes healthier skin, helps maintain a healthy GI tract, helps maintain healthy arteries, and helps improve mild memory problems associated with aging.
Source: Wal-Mart
Cost: $2.43 for 250 tablets, or less than 1 cent per day.

Acetyl L-Carnitine, 800 mg, anyone concerned with living longer and healthier.
Use: Cell health throughout your body, which has a beneficial effect on aging.

Alpha Lipoic Acid, 400 mg,
Use: Excellent free radical fighter; use along with Acetyl L-Carnitine for cell health.
Source: Wal-Mart
Cost: Buy both of these in combined form, at Wal-Mart, which has capsules of Acetyl L-Carnitine 400 mg and Alpha Lipoic Acid 200 mg. Taking 2 of

these each day will satisfy the dosage suggestion. This combination is $7.96 for 30, good for 15 days, or 53 cents a day. This is expensive, but worth it, especially to oldsters like me.

Juvenon, a combination of Acetyl L Carnitine and Alpha Lipoic Acid that can be used by anyone. Juvenon is called *a new anti-aging discovery . . . the first safe, real, anti-aging formulation in our lifetime.*

Use: This is the replacement for the combination Acetyl L Carnitine and Alpha Lipoic Acid discussed in the previous paragraph. However Juvenon also contains biotin, calcium, and phosphorus, resulting in an energy-generating, age-fighting combination that has received worldwide coverage.

Source: Juvenon, Inc. P O Box 432, Manteno IL 60950-9910, 1-800-806-9890, www.juvenon.com.

Cost: 12 bottles (a year's supply) for $199.75, or about 66 cents per day; 6 bottles for $119.85, a little over 66 cents per day; or 3 bottles for $79.90, a little over 88 cents per day.

Comment: This is only slightly more expensive than the combination that I get from Wal-Mart. It also has some additional ingredients that work with the 2 major ingredients, and therefore it might be more effective and convenient for you. On sober reflection, I think my next buy will be Juvenon.

Curcumin, 400 Mg, one capsule daily with food, everyone who is conscientious about their diet and wants to live a long, enjoyable life.

Use: Curcumin has multiple health benefits, including a reduction of inflammation, maintenance of a healthy lipid profile, enhanced bowel and joint functions, maintenance of healthy platelet (blood cells) functions, inhibiting histamine release which results in less sniffling, watery eyes, and the rescue of islet cells in the pancreas. Curcumin also protects against estrogen-mimicking chemicals, protects against free radicals, and promotes normal cell growth. Curcumin effects are **MAJOR** in the body.

Source: The only source I would recommend now is Life Extension Foundation (http://www.lef.org/). Their version is called Super Bio Curcumin, and it is about 7 times more bio-available than Curcumin from other sources.

Cost: The Super Bio-Curcumin from Life Extension is $30.00 for each bottle, but is $19.88 per bottle when a member buys 4 bottles. This works out to about 33 cents a day.

Advanced Supplements

If you have reached your limit with the above supplements and want to do more, then there are a few added supplements to consider. On the theory that every thing helps toward a better and longer life, here they are.

Resveratrol, 50 to 250 mg, everyone past about age 50

Use: This is a workhorse antioxidant, found naturally in red grapes. But get what you need as a supplement (otherwise you would need to drink many bottles of wine per day, not such a bad idea for some people). Resveratrol has many benefits, including improved insulin sensitivity, enhanced mitochondrial function, and reduced expression of inflammatory factors. Resveratrol is being looked at closely right now for its anti-aging abilities, rather important to people like me.

Source: One source is Vitamin World (http://www.vitaminworld.com/); another that I know of now is Renaissance Health. They have a product named Revatrol that you can order via phone (1-866-482-6678) or via the Internet (http://www.revatrol.com/order4/RV0408). Still another source for Resveratrol is Life Extension Foundation (http://www.lef.com/).

Cost: 6 boxes of Revatrol (a 6 month supply) for $179.95, or about 10 cents a day; a 3 month and a 1 month supply is also available at slightly higher cost per day. If you call and you have a spouse that you want to include, ask about the Marriage Proposal deal. The Life Extension version recommended is called Optimized Resveratrol, contains 250 mg, and costs $46.00 per bottle for a non-member, or $34.00 for a member. If you buy 4 bottles, the member price reduces to $31.00 per bottle, or about 51 cents per day.

Additional Factor: Resveratrol is so new that the proper dosage has not been determined yet. Resveratrol from Life Extension Foundation is 20 mg or 100 mg, and Optimized Resveratrol is 250 mg. My little reading on this convinced me to switch to the 250 mg version from Life Extension.

For additional data on Resveratrol, please see Appendix 5.

Glutathione, 600 to 1800 Mg of N Acetyl Cystine (NAC), which is converted to Glutathione in the body.

Use: Glutathione is a master molecule in the body, necessary for many body functions. It is extremely hard to supplement, though. Taking it by mouth in capsules or pills of any kind does not work; acids in the stomach and intestines destroy it. Injections of glutathione also do not work very well; enzymes in the blood also destroy most of it. Instead, NAC is taken in pill form, and this is converted in the body into Glutathione.

Source: One source for NAC that I know of is Vitamin World in Rockvale Outlets http://www.vitaminworld.com/.

Still another method of supplementing Glutathione is a cream containing Dipalmitoyl Glutathione and called Protect 120, which is now available from a special source, Stem Cell Products, 3350 Palm Center Drive, Las Vegas NV, http://www.stem120.com/. You simply rub about an inch-long ribbon of this cream on your upper arm each day.

Cost: $19.99 for 120 600 Mg capsules, or about 17 cents per day for taking the 600 Mg dose of NAC. If you can afford it and you are an oldster like me, take as much as 1800 Mg per day, for an increased cost that you can figure out.

The cost of the Protect 120 is expensive, on the order of $60 per tube. A tube lasts for almost a month, though, so this might not be expensive to you.

For additional data on Glutathione, please see Appendix 6.

Astaxanthin. One 4mg softgel each day

Use: Astaxanthin is a premier antioxidant. This means that it is a very important part of your body defenses, and should be used by everyone who reads this report. Astaxanthin is therefore a **MAJOR** player; I have it in my supplement bag, and so should you.

Source: This is available from Jarrow Formulas, P O Box 35994, Los Angeles, CA 90035-4317, www.jarrow. com.

Cost: A bottle of Astaxanthin containing 60 softgels is $15.95 for me and retails for $21.95. Since the bottle will last about 60 days, this is therefore about 37 cents per day;.

Human Growth Hormone (hGH), 1 packet each day for 5 days, skip two days and repeat. Continue this pattern for 3 months, skip a month, then repeat the entire pattern. Needed by everyone over about 35 who wants to continue to have the best health in life.

Use: hGH is used literally in every cell in your body and washes away the effects of aging. It is currently the ultimate antiaging medicine. Using it, the immune system is revitalized, heart attack and stroke risk factors are diminished, emphysema patients find their oxygen intake improved (they can breathe easier), osteoporosis is prevented, wrinkled skin is restored to youthfulness, sexual vitality is restored, hair color is restored, brain shrinkage is stopped, skin is restored to a more supple and thicker form, and much more. Just think about what it would be like to be 20 to 30 years younger; all your lost energy, ambition, and carefree life. You can now have that return to a more youthful life via hGH.

Source: The only source I would presently recommend is Institute for Vibrant Living (www.ivlproducts.com), P O Box 3840, Camp Verde AZ 86322, phone number 1-800-218-1379. Their version is called Secretagogue hGH Plus; it stimulates the release of hGH from the body's storehouse in the pituitary gland. Another source of an hGH releaser is Goldshield Direct, P O Box 20749, West Palm Beach FL 33416-9963, 1-800-232-3536. Their version is called Premier HGH. It is similar to the Secretagogue hGH product in that is in a packet that you dissolve in water, then drink.

Cost: For the Secretagogue hGH product, the cost is $299 for 6 boxes with 2 additional boxes thrown in, enough for 8 months, or a little over a dollar per day. For someone who is within 20 years of their last day and wants to enjoy those 20 years, this could be well worth it.

Probiotics, No set dosage.

Use: If you have ever had a session with diarrhea or constipation, or consistent gas or bloating, then there is relief available. This relief is known as Probiotics, and it comes in a BB size beadlet or caplet that will survive your stomach acids and do its work in your intestines.

Source: If you are in a hurry or you are just beginning in Probiotics, pick up a packet of Lactobacillus Acidophilus at Wal-Mart or other drug store. This will serve as a starter packet in your quest for good Probiotics. A better version is Probiotic Advantage from Healthy Directions (www.drdavidwilliams.com); their version contains 10 of the most beneficial bugs or flora in beadlets. Still another source is the Institute for Vibrant Living (www.ivlproducts.com), P O Box 3840, Camp Verde AZ 86322, phone number 1-800-218-1379. Their version is called Vibrant Flora 15/50, and contains 15 of the most beneficial bugs in beadlets. If I were buying now, this is the version I would get; I like the company, and it has the most content.

Pyroloquinoline Quinone (PQQ), one 10 mg capsule each day.

Use: PQQ is for everyone of any age that wants to help their mitochondria regenerate and provide a better life. PQQ is the only substance known that will repair and even regenerate your mitochondria.

Source: The only source for PQQ that I am currently aware of is Life Extension Foundation (http://

www.lef.org). Their product is called PQQ Caps with BioPQQ.

Cost: My cost was $59.40 for 4 bottles of 30 capsules each, or 4.9 cents per day. This is minimal.

Irvingia, 150 Mg, one capsule twice daily, everyone who is obese and wants to shed some serious pounds.

Use: For anyone of any age that wants to shed more than 50 pounds in a relatively short time, such as a few months.

Source: The major source for Irvingia that I would recommend is Life Extension Foundation (http://www. lef.org). Their name for the recommended product is Integra Lean Irvingia, which has almost nothing in it except for the active ingredient, Irvingia.

Cost: The Integra Lean Irvingia from Life Extension is $56.00 per bottle for non-members, and $36.00 per bottle if a member buys 4 bottles. This works out to about $1.20 per day, which is expensive, but not to an obese person who is looking for a viable alternative to dieting or other weight-reduction options.

Alkaline Body Ph Balance, no dosage

Use: I am told by several sources that the body Ph (acid balance) should be neutral or alkaline, 7.0 or above on the alkalinity scale. Since most foods contribute to an acid balance, then I have found a product that might be useful that contributes to an alkaline body.

Source: The single product that I know about and have used is something called Alkaline Body Balance. This product comes in a bottle dispenser that easily allows adding drops into any receptacle, including a glass of tea or a coffee cup. The source I know of is from Health Resources, P O Box 3623, Hueytown AL 35023, 1-800-471-5007. Since this product also contains a proprietary blend of minerals, it might be suitable for adding to the output of a home water purification system.

Cost: You can get a 6 month supply of Alkaline Body Balance for $149.70, which includes 2 free gifts and 2 additional bottles. Normal use of this should stretch the available time to near a year or more.

Comment: I was using this to counteract the effects of going off Nexium. I found that if I did not take the "purple pill" when I was supposed to, then I had a really bad case of heartburn. So I am dosing my tea glass with Alkaline Body Balance, and so far it seems to be working. It remains to be seen if the heartburn will eventually go away. After a few weeks, it seems that the heartburn is going away, but it is slow. I recently had a bad couple of nights where it seemed that heartburn was going to overwhelm my defenses; this resulted from a single meal of a Chef's Salad with Bleu Cheese dressing, which is sour but tasty. I used Body Balance to add to my tea, which barely did compensate for the sour Bleu Cheese.

If this is interesting or pertinent to you, please contact me for further detail. This is apparently an on-going situation.

Psyllium Fiber, no dosage

Use: If your diet naturally contains enough fiber that you are regular with your bowel movements (no straining, at least once a day), then you probably do not need a fiber supplement. However, if you are eliminating in small balls or have to strain to eliminate (constipated), then there is probably a good supplement that can "help with" that.

Source: The fiber supplement that I was using is Konsyl, a 100% Psyllium fiber, available at Wal-Mart. I mix about a full tablespoon into my bowl of hot oatmeal for breakfast and it has smoothed out my problems.

Another source for fiber is Metamucil, which you can get in several flavors. My canister is Orange flavored, and I mix a heaping tablespoon into my hot oatmeal every morning. And I like this better than Konsyl; it mixes easily, does not clump up in the microwave, and in general is an easier product to use.

Cost: Minimal. A single container of Konsyl will last me several months. Metamucil is similar in price; one container lasts for several months.

Testosterone, every male past the age of about 50 who wants to get back some of their youthful energy, vim and vigor.

Use: For all the elder generation that wants more zip in their life, including their sex life.

Source: I have been taking Androgel, a Testosterone-containing gel that I rub onto a shoulder each morning; this accounts for part of my vim and vigor. This is available only by a prescription, though, so it is not appropriate for everyone; I have a prescription plan available that lets me economically do this.

I recently became aware of another source of a Testosterone-booster called T-Boost from Renaissance Health, 925 S. Federal Highway, Suite 500, Boca Raton, FL 33432, 1-866-482-6678, www.t-boost.com/order18/tbc040901A. A 6-month supply is available for $169.95; orders for a 3 month supply or a 1 month supply are also available.

Still another source of a Testosterone-booster is TosterAll from Hampshire Labs, 4832 Park Glen Road, Minneapolis, MN 55146, 1-800-279-5517, www.hampshirelabs.com. A 3-month supply is $119,95 plus $7.95 S&H, which gives you an additional 3 months free.

Supplement Recommendations

The recommendations given below on specific health problems are offered in the spirit of help; they help to interpret the data given in the main section above.

Please keep in mind that this section represents my own considered opinion, based on a rather wide reading of available literature. In most cases, I cannot cite a source for many of the statements given; the sources are wide spread and not subject to ready quote.

If you have a problem with what I am saying, then please refer to your own health care provider. And if you do not like what he/she tells you, you may want to find yourself another doctor.

Heart Attacks

In studying cancer statistics, one striking feature showed up. A very high percentage of those people having heart attacks had no discernable reason for the heart attack; their blood pressure was normal, and cholesterol and other risk factors were within their normal ranges. They were apparently in their prime, health wise.

A very big cause of this anomaly has been identified as inflammation, which can be a low level and not discernible to the individual. Such inflammation can result from stress, pressure on the job, or any other mental or physical effort that puts a strain on the system.

Several of the supplements act to reduce inflammation, thus preventing a lot of heart attacks. See Fish Oil, Vitamin D3, aspirin, Curcumin, and Resveratrol.

Congestive Heart Failure

In this failure mode, only Fish Oil and CoQ10 are recommended as really being necessary as preventatives.

But also see Vitamin D3, aspirin, and Curcumin for added benefits.

Fish Oil and CoQ10 are specifically recommended for this condition. Please see Dr. Sears book, The Omega Rx Zone, where he describes several cases of near-death patients that he treated with high-dose pharmaceutical grade fish oil and they recovered.

For anyone subject to congestive heart failure, my recommendation is to take 6 of the Super Omega 3 Fish Oil capsules from Life Extension each day. If you are farther advanced in the disease than this, or if this dosage gives you objectionable gas and/or bloating, then please call Sears Lab, take their advice, and proceed from there (see the fish oil section for access information). Or investigate the krill oil option also discussed in the fish oil section.

Anti-Aging Supplements

If you like and enjoy your present life, then you should plan to extend it as far as it can be and still be enjoyable. For this purpose, you can presently take several supplements that will extend your life. I strongly believe that I am now a typical representative of this group, and therefore what I am taking is what you should be taking. Please see Fish Oil, CoQ10, Vitamin D3, Acetyl L Carnitine/Alpha Lipoic Acid/Juvenon, Resveratrol, Human Growth Hormone, and Testosterone (this last is for men only).

Quality of Life Enhancements

This discussion is specifically applicable to people older than about 50. If you simply want to get your life back into some semblance of enjoyable, then several options are available. Please see Fish Oil, CoQ10, Vitamin D3, Vitamin B-12/Folic Acid, Acetyl L Carnitine/Alpha Lipoic Acid/Juvenon, Curcumin, Resveratrol, Human Growth Hormone, and Testosterone (this last is for men only).

Supplement Sources

One major source of supplements that I use is Life Extension Foundation (http://www.lef.org/. You can become a member, after which your cost of supplements decreases. Membership costs $75 per year, but for this you get a 1665 page tome titled Disease Prevention and Treatment, a yearly subscription to Life Extension Magazine, and almost daily information tips via email. I print out each tip that is interesting and file them. If interested, call 1-800-544-4440; they might "cut you a deal" on the membership fee. In my own mind, the Disease Prevention and Treatment tome itself is almost worth the member fee. It is a major source of information on all kinds of supplements.

Another source of supplements and other vitamins is Dr. Whitaker's Forward Nutrition (http://www. drwhitaker.com/, Natural vitamins from the doctor you trust. You can sort through their catalog to determine if you are interested. Call them at 1-800-722-8008 to order anything or to request a catalog.

This source is not my first choice, primarily because I was exposed to Life Extension first, and in addition Suzanne Somers in her book *Breakthrough, Eight Steps to Wellness,* says that she trusts that Life Extension will provide quality supplements and that what they say is not all hype. That is worth quite a bit to me; I will stay with Life Extension for the majority of my non-Wal-Mart supplement buys. I still sort through their catalog, though; I do NOT buy everything they sell.

The Paradise of Dreams

There are times when I think, when that lone night-light
*   gleams,*
That this world would be better if run as in dreams.

This old world would be great, one big wonderful ball,
If that dog "morning after" didn't happen at all.

And at Spring-cleaning time, without thinking I'd know
That I'll need this next month and won't suffer that woe.

Before buying my wife a small trinket or gift,
I'd know whether she'll like it or be highly miffed.

Phil Sumner

I would know when I'm shopping that I can rely
On the clerk finding me when I'm ready to buy;

When discussions involve subjects deep and obscure,
I would instantly learn them and always be sure.

When the door or the phone demands an answering trot,
I would know who it is and that this time I'm not.

When I want anything, I'd have nothing to chase—
I would know where to find it, any time, any place.

Yes, I think I would like these, they'd be such a boon;
But I'll bet they won't happen—not any time soon!

Chapter 2
Exercise

EXERCISE IS A major key to a longer and more happy life. Just walking at a fairly fast clip for a half hour or so 3 or 4 times a week will pay tremendous benefits. One quote sums up the present attitude of medical professionals. "Regular physical activity is probably as close to a magic bullet as we will find in modern medicine," says Dr. JoAnn Manson, chief of preventive medicine at Harvard's Brigham and Women's Hospital. "If everyone were to walk briskly 30 minutes a day, we could cut the incidence of many chronic diseases by 30 to 40%."

The importance of exercise cannot be over emphasized. The *Use it or lose it* dictum applies here. Don't do it, and say bye-bye to the world, probably prematurely. Do it, and all kinds of good things will happen; you will sleep better, think more clearly, live longer and better, and look at things more kindly. Guaranteed that you will like it!

Exercising some is good, exercising more is better; exercising as little as an hour each week will pay tremendous benefits. Naturally, if you can do more, the benefits will be greater. There is an upper limit to the benefits, but most of us (including me) will never reach it.

It has been recently reported that even exercise in bed counts toward an exercise goal. And this sure beats the treadmill or dumbbells.

Recent studies emphasize the value of exercise and a balanced diet. One study group of 11 men was obese, walked every day at a mild-to-moderate pace for 45 to 60 minutes, and ate a balanced diet high in grains, fiber, vegetables, and fruits. The study results were: a) the men lost 4 percent of their body weight; b) at the start of the study, 7 of the 11 men had hypertension, while at the end of the study none of them did; c) blood pressure dropped by an average of 14 percent; d) oxidative stress, which is the presence of harmful oxygen-free radicals that attack cells and tissues, dropped by 28 percent; e) nitric oxide availability, which helps relax the blood vessels thus reducing blood pressure, rose by 28 percent; f) cholesterol deceased by 19 percent; g) insulin levels dropped by 46 percent; and h) blood glucose or blood sugar fell by 7 percent.

Another study of 7,500 women found that exercisers had a 48% lower death rate from all causes. Still another study found that exercise has beneficial effects on cholesterol; even though the total level of cholesterol did not change, fewer of the HDL (bad) and more of the

LDL (good) particles were formed. Exercising helps you in every way there is, health wise.

According to an article in *Parade* dated January 18 2009, exercise will also benefit your brain. Any exercise that leaves you breathless can have a positive effect on mental operation and on mental plasticity, or the ability for new growth and development. Exercise is not a cure for Alzheimer's and it won't stop you from getting older, but it might help you stay sharper, longer. Don't let age slow you—or your mind—down.

Recent studies seem to show that just the act of trying to help yourself with exercise and health items might help you live longer. It is certain that you will like your life better after trying, and it might be that this is also what makes things better.

This discussion is specifically tailored for seniors (I am one), but other people can use the same procedures with very good results.

Equipment Required

The equipment required for exercising is pretty simple. It consists of: 2 hand springs or small foam or rubber balls for hand exercises; 2 light dumbbell weights, 2 lb (women) or 5 lb (men); and stairs if your house has them or a small 2-step hand ladder used for accessing high places like kitchen cabinets over the refrigerator.

If you can go beyond this minimal set of equipment and do strength training with weights or a treadmill or other suitable exercise device, then you will derive additional benefits. This is the only place that I know of where more is definitely better, short of actually injuring yourself. Again, if in doubt, talk to your doctor.

General or Warm-Up Exercises

Standing or sitting, take several deep breaths. Stretch your body by twisting and bending it several ways; one excellent way is to use your hands and arms and "reach for the sky". Reach as high as you can. Bend forward, backward, and to each side.

Standing with your arms down at your sides, twist your body 90° left then back, and twist it 90° right then back. Repeat this procedure several times, until you feel tired. Repeat with your arms out and free-swinging.

Walk in-place; lift each leg and put it down in the same place. Continue to walk in place until you are tired.

Other suggestions for easy exercises—Walk to the post office if it is within 3 blocks, or whatever greater distance is comfortable for you. When grocery shopping, deliberately take the cart through all the aisles, even though you don't intend to buy anything from some of them. Join the mall-walkers, who gather at a local mall each week. Park a few blocks away from your usual spot, and walk the rest of the way. Use the entrance furthest from your desk at work. Use the bathroom on a different floor. Walk at the airport while waiting. Walk over to talk to colleagues instead of using email or the telephone.

Avoid drive-through windows. Take hikes in a local park. Use the stairs, not the elevator or escalator. Get off the bus one or two stops early and walk, both ways. Rake the leaves or mow the lawn. Go dancing instead of to the movies. Ride a bike instead of taking the car. Take every opportunity to walk to where you want to go instead of using a car, bike, bus, or scooter.

Hand and Arm Exercises

Compress each hand spring or foam ball, hold for a count of 5, then release. Repeat until your hands are tired.

Holding the dumbbells with palms up (forward), bend your arms at the elbows and curl the weights up to a horizontal position. Hold this position for about 1 second, then lower your arms. Repeat this procedure 10 or 20 times, or until your arms are tired. Then turn the weights so that your palms are down (backwards) and repeat the procedure until your arms are tired.

Holding the dumbbells with palms up (forward), raise your arms from the shoulder and bring your straight arms forward and up horizontally. Hold this position for about 1 second, then lower your arms. Repeat this procedure 10 to 20 times, or until your arms are tired.

Holding the dumbbells with palms toward your body, lift your arms from the shoulder and raise your straight arms out to the sides. Hold this position for about 1 second, then lower your arms. Repeat this procedure 10 to 20 times, or until your arms are tired.

Holding the dumbbells with palms toward your body, depress your arms from the shoulder, raising them behind you; bend forward at the same time. Hold this position for about 1 second, then lower your arms. Repeat this procedure 10 to 20 times, or until your arms are tired.

Leg Exercises

Using the stairs or small ladder, step up 2 steps, then step back down. Repeat this several times, then switch the first leg and repeat again. Repeat until you are tired.

Walk in place in your own home or apartment. Just go through the motions of walking while you are standing still. You can even speed things up slightly and simulate jogging this way.

Do any of the walking exercises mentioned above at least once a day. This could be walking the dog, shopping at the mall, or whatever gives you pleasure or purpose. Try to walk for at least 30 minutes each day, spaced out over the day. If you have already accumulated this much exercise in a day, then doing more will help more. Remember that more is definitely better, short of actual damage to your body.

Motivation

If you need motivation to stay interested in exercising, then consider some or all of the following suggestions. Find a partner to exercise with; it is easier to stay interested if another person is involved. Make exercise a priority in your life; add it to your calendar or planner. Don't look at the scale; you are concerned with healthy living by exercising, not in how much you weigh. Wear comfortable clothes, ones in which you can "let it all hang out". Listen to music that you like while exercising; happy tunes are especially appropriate. Chart your progress in terms of the number of repetitions you can do or the miles (blocks, minutes) that you walk, etc. This way, you can evaluate yourself occasionally; an increase in your abilities is a very satisfactory happening.

These exercises are minimal and should cause no problems. An interesting variation can be introduced; count the repetitions in each exercise, and keep a record of this. You should find your count increasing; you should also feel better, more energetic, more in tune with the world. You can also switch to something either more or less energetic, whatever suits your specific needs.

Summary

Are you ready to start living longer and enjoying life more, sleeping better, increasing your endurance and strength, improving your balance to prevent falls, and protecting your bones? Then exercise! Add years to your life; add life to your years!

REVERIE

That old moth-eaten chair
That I napped in for years,
    To me comfy, to them just a blight . . .

Was replaced, I despair—
Please excuse the tears—
    Now I can't sleep, even at night . . . .

Oh, my God! Hear my prayer
As this memory sears,
    And as doleful grows hearing and sight,

Let me remember the air,
Hear a hundred young cheers,
    See the cities all haloed with light,

Smell the flowers, though bare,
Scratch old Bozo's long ears,
    Feel the rain to recall sheer delight,

See the lakeside so fair,
Live a thousand more here's,
    See the geese once again in pure flight . . .

All of these with no fears,
As the end for me nears . . .
    My days then were all sunny and bright . . .

Chapter 3
Life Adjustments

WOULDN'T IT BE wonderful to have good health all the time? To not worry about colds or flu or any other diseases that might be going around? To know that, short of some fatal disease or accident, we had the expectation of living past 90? Or 105 (in a very few years)? Or 150 (by 2050)?

There are many things you can do for yourself to enhance your health and therefore your enjoyment of life, and also extend the enjoyable portion of your life. The more you can assume of the responsibilities for your future, the better off you will be. And isn't a longer, more healthy, and more enjoyable life worth setting as a major goal? My life adjustment recommendations follow:

Take charge of your own health. Learn all the drug names you are taking now, their dosage levels, and what they are for. If you have any doubts about the purpose, activity, possible side effects, or any other characteristics about any drug you are taking, ask your doctor. If you cannot get the information you need from him/her, look for it on the Internet at http://www.google.com/. Type in the drug name, and click Search. You will get a list of possible sites that you can simply click to go there. If you go to a site and it does not have what you want, click the back button on your browser and try again. You should eventually get a description of the drug and its characteristics. And it should be in language that you can understand. Another good source for medical information is http://www.medlineplus.gov/. Still another is **http:www.medinfo.co.uk**, a site in Great Britain that might be helpful. If you still cannot find what you are looking for, try another search engine such as AltaVista or Ask Jeeves.

Review your drug list with your doctor. Eliminate drugs on this list where you can, but don't go against the advice of your doctor. If you absolutely don't like your doctor's advice, find yourself another doctor. You absolutely need one to work with.

Think positive. All kinds of good things will result if you always think positively about life, health, friends, etc. Positive thoughts lift your spirit, invigorate your immune system, and literally improve your health. In one estimate, having a positive attitude can extend a person's life by 7.5 years. So always be cheerful (ABC).

For ordinary cuts and abrasions, don't even go to the doctor. Instead, use an antibiotic ointment (I have had excellent results with Neosporin) and band aids. And if the sight of blood really gets to you, enlist the help of someone else in the family, or the next door neighbor. Otherwise, learn to tolerate blood. If this still leaves you in doubt as to what you can do and how, then check in your community to see if there are any classes being given on **first aid**. Take at least one class, and volunteer for any hands-on exercises.

I am not really advocating the pioneer way of life here, but if it helps you think positively about your own abilities, then think that way. Your first line of defense is you and what you can do.

For viral diseases such as colds and the flu, don't bother going to the doctor unless your temperature is also high. Instead, stay home and take care of it. The doctor can only offer moral support for this, but your spouse and/or children should be able to supply that. Do not in any case ask for or demand an antibiotic from your doctor; antibiotics are worse than useless against viruses. Remember, the bugs are learning; *don't teach them anything more than you have to*. Instead, boost your immune system by taking supplements listed in the Medical Supplements section, especially Vitamin D3.

There are now some anti-viral drugs available via prescription that can shorten the flu misery by about a day and might alleviate the depth of the misery. Whether these are useful to you is very much up to you. If your situation, job, or some other need demands that you be at the top of your form at all times, then talk to your doctor. And stay away from others who have the flu or colds.

There is another possibility for reducing the "miseries" associated with colds; take 1000 mg of Vitamin C each day during the cold. The Vitamin C acts to reduce blood histamine levels, which reduces histamine-caused reactions like a runny nose, itchy, watering eyes, and sneezing.

It has now been proven that chicken soup really is good for colds and the flu. It does reduce the miseries associated with these, and helps speed recovery. So enjoy!

If you are currently concerned about getting the flu, then you should consider getting a flu shot at your doctor's office or other source. This is especially true for seniors older than about 60, and it is also true for individuals of any other age older than about 5 if you have any doubts about your ability to withstand the flu. In addition, if you are in the age range of 5 to 49, you might also consider a new option; the doctor can squirt something called Flu Mist up your nose. It is reportedly just as effective as a shot, but it is less painful and more expensive.

Medical authorities have recently realized that heart attacks and heart disease can also be caused by an inflammation somewhere in the body. Evidence is now apparently overwhelming that this is true; almost half the heart attacks occurring during the last few years have happened to people who had their cholesterol under control, had normal blood pressure, and had no other overt symptoms that would indicate heart trouble.

A simple test will indicate whether an inflammation is in progress anywhere in the body. This test checks for the presence in the blood of a chemical called C-reactive protein (CRP), normally used by the body to fight inflammation. CRP is the body's defense that rushes to heal a cut, burn, or any other injury.

Recent studies show that the level of CRP rises with age, which may be a major cause of the debilitation that normally occurs as we grow older. I am very interested in this one.

Guidelines for how to handle this new information were issued in early 2003; these will eventually filter down through your doctor to you. At present, the guidelines recommend testing only those people who are at risk and are not already being treated. However, if you think you are at risk for heart disease or a heart attack, you should ask for this test. Then let your doctor decide; if you do not like his decision, you can always find another doctor.

Please note that having an inflammation does not mean you will feel bad or otherwise be aware of it. A low-level inflammation can occur anywhere in the body and be completely masked by an apparently normal and healthy life.

If your stomach can tolerate it, take at least a baby aspirin each day; increase this to a standard 325 mg pill if you have any symptoms of stroke. Aspirin is a significant blood thinner, useful along with Vitamin E as protection against strokes. Recent studies have found aspirin also has value in combating some cancers and serious heart problems like heart disease. But recent data indicates that other NSAIDS like Ibuprofen or Tylenol should not be taken at the same time as the aspirin, or the aspirin will lose its heart-healthy abilities. If you are presently taking one of the NSAIDS for arthritis and would like to switch to aspirin for its heart benefits, talk to your doctor first.

Recent findings indicate that long-term use of aspirin (2 years or more) might provide some protection against Alzheimer's. At least one study showed that such use cut the risk of Alzheimer's about in half. I hereby propose a nomination that Aspirin is a "wonder drug".

Evidence is mounting that actions you can take that would be healthy for your heart also might help prevent Alzheimer's. Specific study results show that the following could help: 1) A reduction of high blood pressure; 2) Eating more fruits and vegetables and less red meat, or a low-fat diet containing vitamins such as A, C, and E; and 3) Exercise, "the nearest thing to a magic bullet in modern medicine". This is another reason for following the vitamin and supplement guidelines given earlier, in Chapter 1.

When you are out in the bright sunshine, protect yourself from the effects of the sunlight. At minimum, this means using a sun screen lotion, with an SPF (sun protection factor) of at least 15 and preferably 30, on all your exposed skin. Also use sun glasses, either prescription or otherwise, that are rated to protect your eyes from the UVA and UVB rays in sunlight. The sun screen is to prevent skin cancer, one of the most deadly forms of this disease, and the sun glasses are to protect against cataracts. Please be generous with the sun screen; recent studies show that most people don't put on enough and wind up with much less protection than they think they are getting. Also re-apply it every 2 hours.

Recent advice on sun protection is to wear clothing that is impenetrable to sunshine; in this thinking, sun screen lotion is just not good enough. Also wear a wide brimmed hat to protect your face and neck.

Another thought is that with the Ozone layer in the atmosphere disappearing, UVA and UVB rays will definitely increase in intensity. This means it is more important now to protect yourself, and its importance will increase as we proceed into the future.

If you are smoking, quit. I know this is hard to do; I smoked for many years and was smoking up to 2.5 packs a day. I tried repeatedly over several months to quit, without any success. Then the straw that finally allowed me to quit (about 30 years ago now) was that I thought about all the other things I could buy with the money I was paying out for cigarettes. *You* can quit. I *know* it. And you *will* quit, if you really *want* to. **Make it worth while to yourself, and you will. Your long life health demands it.**

One reinforcer to quitting is that they now know that the very bad effects on your lungs can be reversed after only a very few short years. I was diagnosed with emphysema about 30 years ago, and it has disappeared. And I am still here, which I almost certainly would not be if I had not stopped smoking.

An additional reinforcer is that in a recent estimate, a pack of cigarettes a day costs up to $1190 per year on average; it is more than that in states that have a high tobacco tax, and would be twice that, $2380, if you smoked 2 packs a day. Or, in my case if I were still smoking 2.5 packs a day, it would be $2975 per year, or $248 per month. To calculate what you or your loved one spends, go to http://www.ashline.org/ and try out their smoker's calculator. You will be stunned.

Don't drink alcohol except in moderation, and even then mostly red wine. They now know that alcohol, in moderation, has a positive influence on the heart and on general health. Red wine has some added ingredients that are helpful. The major ingredient in red wine is Resveratrol, which turns on sirtuins, enzymes that help repair cells and perhaps extend life. For a more complete discussion of Resveratrol, see Chapter 1 and Appendix 5.

Some very recent news is that seniors (over 65) should be more careful about taking alcohol. Present recommendations are that a woman take only one alcoholic drink per day, and a man take no more than two drinks. As with everything else medical, talk to your doctor if you have any doubts whatever.

Set regular hours for sleep (8 hours minimum for most people) and see that you get them. Don't short-change yourself; getting less sleep than you need can cause very bad problems. There are apparently people who can live very comfortably on less than 8 hours, but be very sure that *you* can if you get less than 8. It is now recognized that adequate sleep is vital to a healthy heart; for example, study results show that people who get 5 hours or less of sleep nightly are 45% more likely to develop heart disease.

Learn the Relaxation Response, and use it daily. If you have time for it, use it twice a day, just after rising in the morning and then in the evening. At other times of the day, consciously relax all the unused muscles when you are at rest or not otherwise occupied. After a little practice, you can even use the Relaxation Response while jogging or doing any other repetitive exercise. This Relaxation Response is described as follows:

- *Pick a focus word, prayer, or short phrase that is firmly rooted in your belief system. Use the "faith" that will allow you to believe the strongest, that will allow you to wholeheartedly believe. If you are a devout Christian, Jew, Muslim, or any other religious person, then use appropriate words for that faith. If you do not have a religious belief, then use appropriate words such as "Let it be" or "1 2 3 123" or literally anything. The purpose of this focus word or words is to help you ignore the outside world.*

- *Sit quietly in a comfortable position. Let your hands rest on a chair arm or in your lap, so that they are completely at rest and comfortable. You can also do this lying down, but the tendency then is to go to sleep. I do it this way anyway; it is good preparation for sleep. Very relaxing.*

- *Close your eyes. At this point, there should be no distractions such as a radio or TV or loud sounds that you cannot ignore.*

- *Relax your muscles. Consciously think this through, so that your arms and legs do not have any residual tension.*

- *Breathe slowly and naturally, and as you do, repeat your focus word, phrase, or prayer silently to yourself.*

Part of this focus can be repeated on inhaling, with the remainder repeated on exhaling.

- *Assume a passive attitude. This means to pay attention to nothing in the outside world. Don't worry about how well you're doing. When other thoughts come to mind, simply say to yourself, "Oh well," and gently return to the repetition.*

- *Continue for 10 to 20 minutes.*

- *Do not stand immediately. Continue sitting quietly for a minute or so, allowing other thoughts to return. Then open your eyes and sit for another minute before rising.*

Practice this technique once or twice daily. Keeping extraneous thoughts away becomes much easier with practice. I suggest doing this just after rising in the morning and in the evening before bed.

If you have a nagging health problem, one that restricts your activities somehow, then think through the situation surrounding the problem. It might be that you can change something to alleviate the problem. Consider my own experiences as a guide only:

1. *Over many years, I gradually became aware of a real problem with my left hip. The joint ached and*

it literally seemed that I might have to have a hip joint replaced, like my older sister. But in thinking about it, I finally realized that I was putting all my weight on the left leg and hip when I got out of a car. I was literally crouched on one leg, then standing up. When I realized that, I changed the way I exit a car. If I can, I put both legs out, then stand up on both at the same time. If I can't get the right leg out, then I still use the left leg, but lean on the door sill so that it takes a good portion of my weight. Since that realization, the left hip problem has gone away.

2. *A couple of years ago, I realized I was having a real problem with my left thumb; the second and third joints from the tip were extremely tender. I virtually lost the use of the left thumb. Any action that resulted in pressure on either joint was extremely painful. Again, I finally realized that I was using the left thumb in an unusual way. When using keyboard commands on my computer, I was using the left thumb to hold down one key while I used a finger to hit the corresponding action key. When I realized that, I stopped using the thumb for keyboard commands. Instead, I now use one finger to hold down the first key, and another finger to hit the action key. My problem went away after a few weeks.*

If you have a problem with stomach ulcers or chronic indigestion, talk to your doctor about the possibility of an infection with H Pylori. This is a bug they did not even know about until about 20 years ago, but one that is easily corrected with an antibiotic. I had the chronic indigestion problem for many, many years, and when the doctors investigated my stomach in search of another problem, they also found and eliminated H Pylori. When I asked the doctor about when and where I caught it, his reply was that most people do catch it; it is very common.

Wash your hands—often! It is now generally recognized that many of the diseases being passed around in hospitals is due to the fact that hospital personnel do not wash their hands often enough. Between the current patient and the last one, a stop at a sink for washing hands is apparently too much trouble. They have recently started providing alcohol gel packs that can be clipped to the uniform, thus making it more convenient for disinfecting the hands.

In the home, the same situation applies. Many cold and flu sessions could be avoided by simply washing your hands more often. And use the soap liberally; scrub it onto your hands for at least 15 seconds, then rinse. While washing your hands, be careful to also clean under the fingernails. This is especially important before eating. Other advice is: a) don't cough into your hands, and if you do, wash them immediately; b) don't sneeze into your hands, for the same reasons; and, c) don't put your fingers into your eyes, nose, or mouth.

Drink iced tea or hot tea, preferably green tea if hot. Always having a pot of hot water for tea, though, is cumbersome, whereas iced tea bought in gallon jugs is always available and very economical (about $2.50 per gallon locally). I strongly believe that drinking tea is the reason my immune system is so strong. In addition, recent news is that tea may strengthen bones, thus protecting against osteoporosis. Tea also contains enough fluorine to protect your teeth; when thinking back, I have not had any real dental problems in many years. I like it! Tea also contains compounds that reduce heart disease and some types of cancer. Tea increases the level of T cells, which produce interferon, a substance that fights disease. Tea even reduces bad cholesterol readings by about 10%.

In a recent study, heavy tea drinkers (about 19 cups per week) were 44% less likely to die after a heart attack. Moderate drinkers (fewer than 14 cups) had a 28% lower death rate.

Do I really need to say more here? Get with it, and turn on to tea! I hereby nominate tea as a "wonder drug", along with aspirin and penicillin, and (a very recent addition, at least in my mind) exercise.

If you are a senior and you have problems getting medical care, then you might want to insist on treatment. As an example, suppose a senior in his/her 70s or 80s has a cataract and cannot use one eye because of it. Or suppose that you have prostate cancer or some other cancer that usually advances slowly. Your doctor might just think that you are so old that any medical treatment probably would not be worth while. But that is a decision that he/she should not be making; you should insist on treatment if you see it as a benefit to the rest of your life. And if he/she still does not agree, find yourself another doctor.

If you are finding problems getting health care, please consider a hypnotist. If you can be hypnotized (not everyone can), then a good hypnotist can help you ignore pain such as for burn treatment, help speed up the healing process, and can relieve asthma and anxiety. Hypnosis can even make warts disappear. Hypnosis can work very well, but is most successful when used by a medical doctor who also is a hypnotist.

If you have friends, cultivate and protect them; if you do not presently have friends, find some and treat them well. Strive to make at least one new friend each day. A true friend can fill the void of many catastrophes, be a sympathetic listener, and otherwise be the person you would most like on your side during any problem. In some ways of looking at things, friends are what life is all about; the sharing of views and actions is priceless. People with strong social networks: 1) Boost their chances of surviving life-threatening illnesses; 2) Have stronger, more resilient immune systems; 3) Improve their mental health; and 4) Live longer than people without social support. A lady in my area that turned 100 recently says that her favorite "hobby" is friends. They really are priceless.

Some ideas about keeping connected to friends are from Reader's Digest:

- *Stop feeling guilty that you can't spend lots of time with old friends, like you did years ago. Do whatever you can to maintain the relationship now; telephone, e-mail, snail (US) mail, etc.*

- *Meet for coffee or an early-morning walk before you start your workday.*

- *Schedule a regular "Friends Time", in which you set aside one weeknight a month or some other regular schedule, to catch up with your buddies.*

- *Invite a friend to share everyday activities you normally do alone, like exercising, doing errands, or going to your kid's soccer game.*

- *Try to be there for key events in your friend's life—weddings, funerals, graduations, etc. Your presence will make a difference.*

Blow your own horn. Don't be afraid to step up to new responsibilities, and don't be afraid to let people know what you can do, without bragging. For many years, I followed the creed that, if I saw something that needed to be done and no one else was doing it, then I picked it up and did it. And this was in spacecraft. I was able to learn all kinds of things this way; e.g., how all the spacecraft subsystems worked, including the command system and the telemetry and data streams.

Believe in yourself. You do not have to feel inferior to anyone. A mental trick that I have used for many years is to tell myself that, no matter who I am matched up with, I am better than they are *in some way*. As an example, they might be the smartest individual in the world or the richest, but I can do physical things better. Or swim. Or say the alphabet backwards. Or literally anything. You are every bit as good as they are. Conversely, they are every bit as good as you are. You are equals! Don't look down or up at them! Instead, have respect for everyone, including the less fortunate *and* more fortunate ones.

Ask questions! Don't ever be afraid of asking questions. It is far better to ask and have people think you are stupid, since someone might then tell you *why* they think you are stupid and thus answer your question. Most of the time it won't work this way, and you will get a lot of straight answers that will help fill out life. *There are no stupid questions!*

It may seem hard to do, but **Think Happy**. Be positive in all your thinking, and project that attitude on to anyone who will listen or watch. For example, whenever anyone asks me "How are you?", a very common greeting, I always answer "Outstanding!". It may not always be completely true, but I get a lot of positive responses from it, and just saying it helps me!

Live every day as if it is your last, that there is no tomorrow. Then one of these days, it will turn out that you are right. But in between then and now, you will have *lived*. And probably *enjoyed the trip*.

Avoid violence and other emotionally involved programs on TV and anywhere else. If you must endure a session like this, take time afterwards for the Relaxation Response exercise discussed earlier in this book.

If not already addicted to music, then become addicted and make it a central part of your life. Listen to it when you are blue or discouraged, especially some bouncy, happy tunes, and I guarantee you will come out of it smiling.

If you can even come close to carrying a tune, strongly consider singing. If you can't hold a tune, sing to yourself so that there will be no criticism; sing or hum along with your favorites to learn carrying a tune. And belt it out! Project! If needed, I'll give encouragement and advice. I think I sing fairly well. At least well enough to enjoy it! Enough said?

Expose your children to music of all kinds. The nursery rhymes are fine for toddlers, then graduate up from there as they grow. It would also help very much if they were exposed to music at school, if they were taught at least the rudiments of notes and how to read them. Music at this stage in life will stay with them the rest of their lives; make it memorable. And kill two birds with one stone; sing nursery rhymes to and with your children. They are only young once; enjoy them.

A fascinating aspect of music is that it might be useful for comatose people in hospitals and nursing homes. Tests were run in an English hospital; a singing group "sang" to the patients without words. The patients reacted to the singing in various ways. Some began slower and deeper breathing. Some made grabbing movements of the hands or turned their head. Some opened their eyes, and some even regained consciousness.

Expose your children to reading. Read to them as toddlers, and teach them to read when they are ready for it. Dr. Seuss is excellent; talk to teachers at school or other parents for other suggestions. If you can somehow "inoculate" your children with a love of reading, then you will have given them something they will have a **major** use for the rest of their lives. In thinking back on my own life, I believe that reading just came naturally with me, and I still very much enjoy a good book, fiction and fact.

But it might have been faster and more complete early in my life if I had had active encouragement. Do *your* children a big favor; teach them to *enjoy* reading (and therefore learning).

Please note that you might need to become involved with books while your children are in school. Present school books have been watered down so much to avoid controversy that they are little better than bland pap. If your schools are not providing an education that includes the classics in literature and thinking exercises in world events, then you probably should get involved with the local PTA and any other influence group such as the school board; attend their meetings and at least ask questions. For an excellent list of good books that your children should be studying, look at *The Language Police,* Appendix 2, by Diane Ravitch.

Somewhat related to reading is another thing that has shaped my life very much. I tell everyone who will listen that I have been going to school every day of my life. I almost never go through a day when I don't learn something. And I really like that. I like to learn just to be learning. Maybe what I learn is just that another tool exists that I didn't know about yesterday; but who knows, I might need that tool tomorrow. I window shop for things like that, and it does not cost me a cent.

If time permits, take a class on any subject you are interested in. Do you like looking at the stars? Take a class on astronomy, possibly available through your local astronomy club. Are you interested in ancient history? Many colleges offer summer courses that could interest you. Taking any class increases your knowledge, expands your mind, and acts as a positive stress reducer.

An excellent source of top flight instructional materials is available from The Teaching Company (http://www.teach12.com/). They have DVDs available on history, physics, astronomy, science and mathematics, fine arts, music, geology, religion, philisophy, literature, and many other topics. If you contact them, they will be happy to send you a catalog of their wares, and probably pester you with future announcements.

Take positive actions to reduce stress. As an example, if you are stopped at a stop light and pressed for time, talk to yourself to avoid being upset. Additional ways to reduce stress are:

- *Try abdominal breathing, which lowers tension levels and promotes relaxation. In one method, lie on your back, place one hand on your abdomen, and concentrate on the movement of your hand as you concentrate on breathing. Raise your hand as far as you can. Naturally, breathe deeply during this process.*

- *Neck and shoulder massage can relieve tension; hot or cold packs on the neck and shoulders also help.*

- *Use progressive muscle relaxation, a systematic technique for reducing muscle tension. Tighten a group of muscles for a few seconds, then relax them and focus on releasing tension and stress. Start with the muscles in the toes and feet, and work upward to your neck and head.*

- *Stretching exercises can relieve tensions all over the body. Stretch while sitting, lying down, or walking. In one scenario, simply "reach for the sky"; this can be used at any time, sitting, lying down, or standing.*

- *A brisk walk of several minutes while thinking relaxing, calming thoughts will release natural pain killers in the brain, producing lowered tensions.*

- *Fairly brisk exercise of any kind that will raise your heart rate will relax your body and provide a calming influence.*

- *Meditation can reduce tensions and stress. See the Relaxation Response procedure earlier in this chapter for an excellent technique. This is highly recommended.*

If you don't have house plants already, bring them into your apartment, house, condo, or wherever you live. Especially in winter, these plants have several very positive influences on our lives: 1) They freshen the air we breathe; they take in carbon dioxide and breathe out oxygen, the very thing we need the most, and especially needed if the house is well insulated and weather-stripped; 2) They provide greenery and color in a world of mostly white and black, thus relieving the monotony; 3) They provide satisfaction and enjoyment for the person doing the work, in getting something to grow; 4) They will reduce stress in everyone in the vicinity who can see their greenery and blooms.

If you want to get into this, talk to your local nursery. Some suggestions that work well for us are: 1) Pandana, easy to grow and propagate to obtain new plants; 2) Rubber tree, easy to grow but requires a large pot (our plant is 4 feet tall and just as wide); 3) Christmas Cactus, easy to grow but slow to bloom, these bloom between Thanksgiving and Christmas and are well worth the time and trouble; 4) Snake Plant, easy to grow and care for; and 5) Sweet Potato, probably the easiest of all, simply put several tooth picks into the sweet potato and suspend it in a container with the bottom of the potato in water, but be warned that it grows via runners that are sometimes more than 6 feet long. Some more exotic plants that could also be considered are: 1) Jade plant, easy to grow and mainly decorative; and, 2) Aloe, the old fashioned source of a healing balm.

You can practice gardening in this way year-round. Cold sensitive house plants can be placed outdoors in the late spring until early fall, then be brought indoors when there is danger of freezing. After spending all summer on our outside deck, our rubber tree plant is a thing of beauty. Likewise, the snake plants, Christmas cactus, and Aloe look very healthy again. The summer sun did wonders!

Another outlet for positive enjoyment that also involves plants is gardening, whether in a true vegetable garden or in some simple flower beds that you coax into life during the summer. There is something positively peaceful about growing things. There is also something positively peaceful about getting rid of plants that you don't want, especially those troublesome weeds. Pulling them out by the handful is an excellent way to relieve some pent-up stress. So, whenever you are feeling up tight, simply rip out some weeds and you will certainly feel better.

For your own safety, peace of mind, and several desirable characteristics, make sure there are trees and other plants of all kinds around you, even if you have to plant them and wait a few years for them to grow. This is true for individual homeowners as well as for apartment complexes. A study of several apartments in Chicago showed that all kinds of crimes were less in those complexes that had trees and other plants.

Another study in Japan has shown that people who live near trees live longer. This included living near parks and tree-lined streets. One theory of this is that living near trees made the people more appreciative, and therefore more active. Another theory is that the increased oxygen level around the trees is beneficial.

One under-appreciated aspect of trees is that they make a hot day more tolerable; a good sized tree will provide the equivalent of several tons of air conditioning. A judiciously planted tree will also block a lot of sunshine in the summer, thus keeping the house cooler. This same tree, if it loses its leaves in the fall, will allow sunshine through in the winter, thus helping with the heating bill.

If you don't have a pet already and do not have allergies or any other reason that would interfere, then seriously consider getting a pet of some kind. Get a large dog if you have plenty of outside room for it to run, a small dog if you have less room or live in a place that requires a leash on pets outdoors, or a cat if you have no outside room at all or don't want to walk them outside. But be sure that the pet is one you want, and one that you will be willing to feed and otherwise care for. For all around utility, I strongly lean toward a very cuddly cat that will jump into your lap and purr until you pet it. A cat litter box and feeding bowls are all it needs, and it can be left in the home for a weekend or even longer, which would allow the owners to take a vacation or stay overnight somewhere else at any time.

Getting the pet from a pet hospital would be good; they should already be spayed or neutered when you pick them up. If you get a kitten, it can be trained to be a petty pet, but its antics as a kitten might be troublesome.

It is now known that a pet, any pet, is a strong stress-reducer. There are cardiovascular benefits (it is good for your heart), and mental health benefits. Your pet may actually help keep you healthy and active, and therefore alive and enjoying it.

There are many organizations now that take pets, dogs and cats mainly, into hospitals where they provide comfort to patients. The almost universal reaction by patients is to smile and to want to pet the pet. The visit of any pet is the high point of their day. There is even an organization that will train you and your pet for visits to hospitals and other places where they would be welcomed. This organization is Delta Society, and they can be reached at 580 Naches Avenue SW, Suite 101, Renton WA 98055, or on the Internet at http://www.deltasociety.org/

Two very good reasons for having pets around children are: 1) It has been found that children who live around two or more cats or dogs before their first birthday are less likely to have allergies of any sort, and 2) Some dogs will "adopt" a child and spend most of its time in the vicinity of the child, I believe to protect it. I have personal experience with the so-called weiner dog (dachshund) with this.

If you have time for it, strongly consider being a volunteer. This does not pay very well money wise, but the pay is phenomenal for the psyche. What you give comes back to you, many times multiplied. Some good suggestions to consider are: 1) For the ladies, be a volunteer at the local hospital; 2) For the men, the local fire department; 3) Mostly for the men but also allowed for the ladies, call Habitat for Humanity, who builds and retrofits housing for lower income families; 4) Either sex, try the local library, who need help with moving things around (mostly books); and 5) If you are in a rough neighborhood, consider joining a neighborhood watch program.

If you still feel like volunteering but none of the above has appealed to you, please consider putting your name in with the USA Freedom Corps, which can be reached at 1-877-872-2677. If you will let them know your skills and your desires, they will almost certainly put you in touch with the people who can use your services.

Help your neighbors, and anyone else who seems to need it. Helping others has been shown to lengthen lives; in one study, people who had helped anyone in the past year were 50% more likely to be alive 5 years later.

Practice forgiveness on a regular basis, in accord with how many people are on your personal hit list. Forgiving others can be very beneficial to your health. I read a very appropriate story recently in Reader's Digest—*At my church one day, a woman who had often snubbed me went out of her way to give me a big hug before the service. I was surprised by her gesture, and wondered what had initiated her change of heart. I got my answer at the end of the service.*

"Your assignment next week", the minister instructed, *"is the same as last week. I want you to go out there and love somebody you just can't stand"*. And this is a perfect illustration of why I think religion will survive, and quite possibly even thrive.

I am reminded of another story I heard recently. A close friend from the place where I worked for many years was always talking about her "mother's other daughter". My friend and her sister were not on speaking terms or any other kind of terms for many years. But they have recently reconciled, and now get together fairly often.

There is a tremendous idea proposed by Ann Landers, of the newspaper personal advice column. She suggests that we designate April 2 as Reconciliation Day. On that day, make a positive effort to mend fences, call that old friend who you haven't talked to for years, say Hi! to all your neighbors, and in general be the original hearty greeter wherever you go. Offer to hug anyone that you think would accept it. Then when this comes easily on April 2, try carrying it to other days. If enough of us do it, maybe the politicians will take heed and really do the country up proud. *As a very good starter for you, do this on the same day you read this paragraph.*

A related thought is appropriate here: *When you praise another person, you make two people happy.*

Consider it a personal goal to have at least one good laugh each day. A real belly laugh, that is. Guaranteed to relax you, relieve stress, help restore your self-confidence, diminish your inhibitions, and contribute to your good health. Watching a comedy show on TV at the end of the day helps many people; outright chuckles over something sent to them via electronic mail (email) helps many others; and even watching the people go by in a supermarket or mall can provide some (very quiet) amusement.

If you have a problem with laughing on a personal or private basis, consider joining a laugh club. Yes, there is such a thing. They were apparently started in India, and there are at least 200 clubs in the good old USA, including one in NYC and another in San Diego. You should adopt their motto about laughing, "Fake it . . . fake it . . . until you make it!" You may not always feel like laughing but if you keep faking it, eventually it will be real. So let's all ABC! (Always Be Cheerful!)

There is a study, now in process, to investigate the connections between laughter and health. Called Rx Laughter, the study will include people of all ages, cultural backgrounds, and economic groups. In addition, Comedy Rx events have benefited many local hospitals and organizations such as Gilda's Club, The Wellness Community, American Cancer Society, Make-a-Wish Foundation, Ronald McDonald House, American Diabetes Association, and March of Dimes. In one quote, "When you're laughing, you can't help but feel better".

An organization that specializes in laughter is the Laughter Heals Foundation. Their stated objective is to bring laughter into hospitals and physical rehabilitation centers; they offer a way to fix broken funny bones.

Laughter has been called one powerful antidote to stress. When you are laughing, you can't help but be cheerful. Laughter can do the same things to the body as beta blockers, and it sure is a lot more fun. So laugh. Again!

One of the most telling studies of the effects of laughter was a 1997 study of 48 heart-attack patients. Half the group watched comedy shows for 30 minutes each day; the rest of the group served as controls and watched nothing. After a year, 10 patients in the control group had suffered repeat heart attacks, compared with only 2 in the group that watched the shows. Again, laugh!

If you are a woman and you "leak" when you laugh too hard, there is probably a good solution for that. Stress incontinence can be treated by exercises of the pelvic floor muscles by repetitive contractions, something called Kegel exercises. If this happens to you, talk to your doctor. If you would like to look this up on the Internet, go to http://www.niddk.nih.gov/, and do a search for Kegel Exercise.

Have you positively cried for joy or uncontrollably blubbered lately, during some musical performance, during some religious sermon, or during the greeting of a long-missing but treasured sibling or friend? If you have, then consider yourself normal and a member in good standing with the human race. Everyone needs to cry for joy occasionally. It happens to me when reading a poignant book like *A Beautiful Mind.*

When you are stopped for any reason, consciously relax all the muscles you are not using. For example, if you are standing, relax your arms and hands. If sitting, relax your arms and legs. Be the original cool cat!!!

Dream. Dr. Martin Luther King is famous for 3 things; 1) he was assassinated, 2) he advocated non-violence, and 3) he gave his "I have a dream" speech. He was so right to have a dream. And so should you be. Dare to dream. Seek out a dream if you don't have one. Adapt or adopt someone else's dream if you can't invent your own. But acquire a dream, however you can, and live it. Assiduously. Dreams will become easier in the future, due to the more relaxed, more laid-back attitudes that will prevail then.

My dream is to live long enough to see many of the things happen that I have described in this book. By staying active and living right (I follow my own recommendations), I hope to achieve 90+. I am totally fascinated by what is happening now, and I want to see where it all goes. I also fully intend to enjoy the trip.

Please remember also that you do not need to have *all* your dreams fulfilled. There have been many cases where the failure to achieve some dream has resulted in the achievement of something better. For example, failure to get into a specific college might let you enter a college that, in retrospect, was the ideal choice for you. So keep your options open; the closing of any door can open many others.

When the blahs have seemingly triumphed over your naturally buoyant nature and nothing seems to help, take a nature walk outside. Take the time to look closely at whatever is in front of you, from ice in the Winter to cherry blossoms in Spring to all the greenery in Summer to the colorful "stuff" available at the roadside stands in Fall. If you look closely enough, there is something of beauty in any scene you can see. One of my personal delights is to go walking during a snow storm in Winter; another is to look at all the ice on trees. And I don't think I need to mention cherry tree blooms or tulips or any of those things. But whatever you do during this sojourn outside, look at everything and enjoy it. And you will return indoors refreshed and maybe ready for another round in the cycle of life.

A young poet named Mattie Stepanek has a couple of concepts that are worth thinking through. One of these is Heartsong, or the ability or purpose that God, or providence, or whatever power, intended for you. Another phrase for this is native ability, or what you naturally can do or learn or achieve. My own Heartsong, for example, is writing technical material; I supported my family for more than 30 years that way, and I have written this book. Heartsong is something each of us should discover about ourselves. And once you discover your Heartsong, make the achieving of it your dream and live it assiduously. There probably will be disappointments and temptations along the way, but keep your dream in mind and return to it when you can.

Another concept by Mattie is that after a storm, we should remember to play. After one of life's bitter surprises, many people hunker down and wait for the next disaster to hit; we should instead be glad, and rejoice! Play! After all, we are still alive, still in relatively good health, and still have oodles of good things to look forward to. And if this is not true of you, think about it, long and hard, and I believe that you will find they really are true of you. Life really is good! We have only to look at it in the right way, and it becomes good!

Subscribe to Readers Digest and read it. It has all kinds of good things between the covers in each issue, including such articles as "Why Doctors Now Believe Faith Heals", May 2001, and departments in every issue like "Everyday Heroes", "News of Medicine", "Laughter", and many more. To me, this magazine is a gold mine that tells me many things I need to know. It will inform you (good). It will make you laugh (good). All the articles are short and sweet (good). And you will enjoy it (good). The News of Medicine column alone is worth the price to me; I need every advantage I can find to keep on living, and things are happening very quickly now.

If you are currently in a job that you absolutely cannot tolerate, then quit and find yourself another job. In fact, consider this strongly if you are simply tired of your present job, its ups and downs, or have a personality conflict with your boss. Life is not worth a thankless job, even if it does put bread on the table. But be sure to find your new job before you quit your old one. Changing into a career that you like or even love is not selfish; it is necessary if you are really going to succeed in life. A brother-in-law of mine stayed in a job like that for more than 20 years, and he had a heart attack and died in his 60s, about a year after he retired.

For a one sentence mantra on life and living: *Work like you don't need the money—Love like you've never been hurt—Dance like no one is watching.*

For another one-sentence mantra on life and living, this one attributed to Mahatma Gandhi: *You must **be** the change you wish to see in the world.*

For another, this one an old Swedish Proverb: *Fear less, hope more; eat less, chew more; whine less, breathe more; talk less, say more; hate less, love more; and all good things are yours!*

For still another: *I don't panic when I get lost; I just change where I want to go.*

For an expression of desirable family traits: *You work hard. You protect and provide for your family. You put your responsibilities before your desires. You lend a hand when someone's struggling, listen and hold a hand when someone's hurting, speak up when someone needs guidance, stand up when the truth needs a friend.*

Of course, the actual health approach you use should be discussed with your doctor. And if he looks sideways at you when you mention some of the topics in this book, ask him if he knows what is being discussed. If he does not, and does not want to know, find yourself another doctor. You **need** a doctor to work with.

I think that our ability to control or to strengthen our immune system will simply add to the benefits gained otherwise. If we are healthier, don't get sick or as often, we will be happier and more contented. I know that I presently am. I very much like life, like living, like doing things like this book, like physical work, like an intellectual challenge, like music, like everything. I have no enemies that I know of, except Father Time, and I stiff-arm him whenever I can. And my fervent wish is that you would join me.

No Comfort!

Our daughter can't wait
For that party at eight,
*   When all of her friends will be near.*

Then it comes—the house whirls
With a group of young girls,
   That act much like a herd of young deer.

The party begins,
With laughs, shrieks and grins!
   It's fun time! It's dance time! It's here!

When that loud hi-fi sound
Seems to crackle and pound
   At full volume, assaulting my ear;

When they're sent out the front
On a Scavenger Hunt
   And the resulting dead quiet seems queer;

When excitement runs high—
"Something's out there!", they sigh—
   Caused by tales of when monsters appear,

And I'm drawn in at 2:00
To sing songs with this crew,
   To settle and quiet their fear;

When I'm wakened at 6:00
By a chant, of all tricks—
   "WE WANT BREAKFAST!" resounds low but clear;

It's no comfort to know,
In the midst of this woe,
*   That the next one is not till next year.*

Chapter 4
Diet

ON A DAILY basis, eat a reasonably balanced diet, mixing green, yellow, and red vegetables, fruits, and some meats with very little fat (but note that you *need* some fat in your diet, which should be vegetable oil, canola oil, olive oil, or some other unsaturated fat). Fish and nuts of all kinds are specifically approved for consumption.

Avoid saturated fats like non-lean bacon and trans fats. The trans fats are listed in many present guidelines. The trans fats are formed when vegetable oils are solidified by a process called hydrogenation; they are presently found in baked goods, processed foods, and fried dishes. Trans fats are doubly bad; they raise bad cholesterol and also lower good cholesterol. If you want to check your current purchases for the presence of trans fats, look for the words "partially hydrogenated" or "hydrogenated". Many of the margarines I look at now have a statement of zero trans fats, but they still have hydrogenated in their contents list. I still steer clear of these; there are now several that do not, so I now have a choice.

The french fries at any current fast food place like McDonalds or Burger King are currently good from a trans-fat standpoint. They have changed the oil that they use for frying things. I still do not indulge in fries very often, though; I don't need the calories.

According to a recent, thorough evaluation of nutrition, the federal diet guidelines should be modified somewhat. Instead of the groupings shown in the Diet Pyramid, the new guidelines may be in percentages, which provides guidance to almost everyone. They might say that people should get about half of their calories from carbohydrates, about one third from fat (mostly unsaturated fats such as fish and nuts), and the rest from protein. They also say that everyone should get an hour of vigorous exercise each day, twice what was previously recommended by the Surgeon General in 1996. This study was commissioned and issued by the Institute of Medicine, who asked the nation's top experts for advice and guidance on fat, protein, carbohydrate, fiber, and other major components of the American diet.

The diet recommendations will probably change to accommodate the new guidelines within a few years. But what form these will take is only partially known. A replacement of the present Diet Pyramid is one possibility, but there are others also. Stay tuned!

Substitute more healthy foods so you can still enjoy old standards. As an example, I still *occasionally* enjoy pie a la mode; but instead of ice cream, I use frozen vanilla bean yogurt. And I like it just as well. And I *really* like fresh strawberries, that have been picked at the top of their sweetness, with frozen vanilla bean yogurt.

If you have a cholesterol problem, the first approach is to control this through diet, via a change in life habits. If this is not completely successful, talk to your doctor about a prescription to control cholesterol. But also be aware that cholesterol medications, known loosely as statins, can have side effects that cause other problems. Keep talking to your doctor.

One of the side effects that statin drugs have is to reduce CoQ10 in the body. For this reason, I quit using a statin drug, and so far my triglycerides are still in line (I am taking the supplements discussed in Chapter 1, and I talk to my doctor).

The Hazards of Modern Living

I'm no absent-minded professor—
Not prone to forget, I argue;
But now and then I catch myself,
Doing things I shouldn't do.

I misplace things in real strange ways,
And lose things in plain view;
And absent-mindedly forget,
The where and when and who.

How else can I account for things
(Except that I just don't think)
Like the dish cloth in the Frigidaire,
The butter in the sink?

Or when the baby cries at night,
And both my shins get barked;
Or waiting for a traffic light,
The car ahead is parked?

Or pouring coffee in the ash tray,
(While busy talking shop),
And stubbing out my cigarette
On the nearby table top?

And many other things like these,
Too numerous to state;
Like the tickets safely back at home,
Us at the ball park gate!

But these small things don't bother me—
I'm worried not one whit;
I don't lose a moment's sleep at night,
O'er the fact that life's a skit.

Phil Sumner

For I've a strong suspicion now,
If you'll be true to me;
Things also happen to you and you,
Just like they do to me.

Chapter 5

The Sumner Weight Reduction Plan

HAVE YOU EVER wanted to reduce your weight? Have you tried some diet plan unsuccessfully, possibly lost weight only to gain it back? Well, there is hope for you; I have a method that costs you nothing, and can help you lose weight the easiest way there is.

There is general agreement that to lose weight, you have to take in less calories; my plan does this in an easy-to-use manner. Nothing magic, just a little self control, and I give ways to help with that.

There are many weight reduction plans in existence; you only have to hear names like Weight Watchers, Jenny Craig, LA Weight Loss, and the Atkins Diet to know that. All of them promise to help you you lose weight, and most of them deliver on that promise if you follow their directions. Unfortunately, however, most of us subsequently regain the weight we so painfully lost.

The major problem with all the diets out there is that you lose weight in a hurry, but there is no provision for keeping the weight off. There is no real support for your new needs, and hunger or habit does you in; you put the weight back on.

If you have had non-success on other diets, then try this plan; the financial risk is zero. I strongly believe that you can reduce your weight to a level you are comfortable with, and thus you will be able to enjoy a more healthful weight and a more enjoyable life.

There is an answer for your significant weight reduction and keeping it off, just as there was for my wife and I. We have successfully lost about 50 and 35 pounds, respectively, and we are now in the process of maintaining our new weight.

The weight-reduction secrets we have used can be summarized very easily. First, take it slow; don't expect, and don't try for drastic results overnight. Instead, shoot for a weight reduction of a pound or so each week, which will let you reach your goal over several months. Second, simply reduce what you eat for breakfast and lunch, and have a normal dinner. Third, exercise as much as you can and feel comfortable doing; this is not an absolute essential, but it helps you feel better as you reduce your weight. And it is absolutely healthful for you. Fourth, occupy your mind with something challenging or anything else that will make you think during this time. Fifth, find ways to enhance your life; make new friends and cherish old ones, find and use new exercises or exercise methods, think positive, enjoy each day as it comes, take any opportunities to learn new things. In other words, be happy and forward-looking. And if you are not basically happy now, find ways to become happy. Is there a pet in your future? A long-postponed vacation? Some other teaser or coveted item?

For breakfast, I switched from cereal and milk to just a small handful of mixed nuts and sometimes a single coconut cookie. For lunch, I switched from a sandwich with cheese and some kind of meat and bread to an apple or orange and a couple of handfuls of potato chips. Then for dinner, I had whatever came along; a 6-inch hoagie (grinder, submarine, whatever you call them locally), a couple of slices of pizza, some microwave dish, or some other normal dinner, which during the summer included sweet corn on the cob. I have now lost about 35 pounds, and I am at about the weight I want to be.

To keep my mind from dwelling on food, I habitually work on something that occupies my mind. Like working on the computer writing things like this book or poetry, reading (a lot, both fiction and non-fiction), music (playing or listening), watching favorite TV shows, adding to a 40 x 28 latch hook rug for a Christmas gift, playing the numbers game Sudoku, learning to crochet, window shopping at WalMart or KMart, helping around the house, and many more. I do *not* lack for things to do. Deliberately. And willingly.

Similarly, my wife has switched from a bagel for breakfast to a bowl of hot oatmeal cereal. For lunch, she switched from a sandwich and fruit to a bowl of yogurt with fruit (both breakfast and lunch are largely carbohydrate free). For dinner, she had the same things I did (naturally). Over a period of about 5 months, she has lost about 50 pounds, and still plans to "lose a few more". To keep herself occupied, she works part-time as a legal secretary, and crochets many of her Christmas gifts and does other needlework. She watches several favorite TV programs, including Bill Cosby, science fiction shows when they are available, Martha Stewart, and antique shows.

You can do the same things that my wife and I did to reduce weight. Simply eat less than usual at breakfast and lunch, and have a normal dinner. And "pig out" occasionally when relatives come visiting or whenever you want to reward yourself, but then return to the minimal breakfast and lunch the next day. After all, your objective is to lose weight long-term, not to torture yourself along the way.

After you get your weight down to where you want it, simply eat a little more at breakfast and lunch, or add mid-morning or mid-afternoon snacks of fruit or some other non-carbohydrate. As an example, I now frequently have a piece of french toast or a pancake for breakfast, and sometimes have an actual sandwich for lunch. In my case, this maintains my new weight. And when my weight shoots up due to dinner out or a buffet breakfast, I simply return to a minimal breakfast and lunch the next day. When I go for a buffet breakfast, where it is "all you can eat", I often skip lunch entirely.

If you plan to reduce your weight, plan to either borrow or acquire a set of scales that you can use at home for monitoring your weight. Then use this daily, at about the same time each day, to check your weight. Record this each time, and check your progress this way. I do believe the steady reduction of your weight will be a satisfactory achievement mark for you. A special note here. Don't worry if your weight bounces up and down a pound or so during the day or day to day; this is entirely normal. It is the long-term weight reduction that you want. Also be sure that your state of dress is the same each time. For example, I apparently carry 7 pounds around during the winter, which results from my clothes, shoes, and the things in my pockets (a man usually has keys, change coins, wallet, and several other items in his pockets). I suggest weighing yourself in the buff, just after getting up and before getting into the shower.

An additional caution. If you go with the steps listed above, you also need to be certain you are getting all the nutrients you need, which is a lot more involved than it was as recently as 20 years ago. For example, be sure to refer to Chapter 1. Talk to your doctor about what you are doing, and ask him for further recommendations. You just might get the pleasant instructions not to lose any more weight. Are you laughing? It happened to me! Which is why I am now holding my weight! From 229 down to 192, I am at a weight that is acceptable to my doctor. Since that was written in 2002, my weight has slowly gone down and is now stable at 181 to 185

This weight reduction plan is revolutionary in several ways. First, it costs you nothing, and in fact your costs will go down slightly due to you not eating as much. Second, there is no special diet, nothing to remember to do or not do. Third, it happens over several months, which allows your body to become accustomed to its new feeding pattern. Fourth, it allows you to binge out on food occasionally, and provides a method for recovering from them. Fifth, once your new diet becomes habitual, you won't miss the old ways; you can then truly enjoy life to a much fuller extent than previously. And you can again wear those clothes that you grew out of.

This weight reduction plan is one that can have a dramatic effect on your life. If you follow these recommendations and successfully lose weight and keep it off for several months or years, it will certainly help you with your self esteem and life happiness. You will like being alive more, and enjoy life more. You just might feel like shouting your happiness to the world. If so, please do.

A special note. This diet plan can be used by anyone, from the mildly overweight to the truly obese. But it is most successful where the desired weight reduction is in the neighborhood of 60 pounds or less. If you want to reduce more, plan on staying with this plan for a longer time, perhaps a year or more. Slow and easy is a **major** part of why it works; this allows the weight reduction to happen, and allows your body to get acquainted with its new requirements.

For you truly obese types, there is some good news medically. A drug called PYY cuts the appetite, resulting in eating about 30% less. The injectable form may be available soon; a pill to do the same thing may be available now. If this is important to you, check with your doctor as to availability and cost.

Still another option for truly obese people is the supplement Inviglia, discessed more fully in Chapter 1.

Chapter 6
Religion

THIS IS A taboo subject in many books, but I think it is proper here. Religion will probably still be with us for the next 50 years, and possibly for the next 1000. There may be less structure in the future (inner city churches are hurting now, in many cases). But churches serve many desirable and needed functions, such as socializing, quality of life reminders (the preacher's sermons), and every day enjoyment. I think they will survive, if only in the form of smaller, more shared churches with more specialized mandates.

I would dearly love to see a merging of the various congregations within the Protestant faiths, and possibly even Protestant with Catholic. I read recently that two major parts of the Protestant faith were in talks to merge. There was also a recent local newspaper article that evangelicals and charismatics (suburban and urban congregations), are considering merging. And a recent news article states that a national alliance of Christian churches was recently proposed. The reason for this was simple, "Both the National Council of Churches and National Association of Evangelicals have undergone financial and organizational woes in recent years."

As for me, I have no religion. I am not a Catholic, Protestant, Jew, Muslim, or any other named religion. Unless you include the religion of life, to which I am very devoted. My reasons for this are really pretty simple. I cannot see how each of the various branches of religion can all claim to be right, that their way is the only way to God. I also fail to see the necessity of God or religion as an explanation of my life; biology and several other current scientific fields as they are now known is sufficient for that.

However, I believe that there is some power that we don't now understand, and that power helps us in many ways. But is that power in each of us? In the mind that we don't completely understand yet? In a very good book, *Discover the Power Within You, A guide to the Unexplored Depths Within,* Eric Butterworth gives very cogent reasoning for his belief that the *force, potential, presence dwelling within us, creator, God,* or whatever you want to call him/her/it, resides in each of us and can be invoked to provide services in our favor.

Another very good book that disusses the power within each of us is *The Power is Within You,* Louise L. Hay. She talks about the *Power, Intelligence, Infinite Mind, Higher Power, God, Universal Power, Inner Wisdom, etc.*

Again, she is talking about a power within each of us that is capable of helping us in many ways.

This book is intended to provide an alternative view of conventional religion. It is not intended as a defense of either religion or non-religion, but instead tries to present an alernative view that you might not have encountered anywhere else, thus making any decsion on your part more solid and set in reasoning.

Reference Books

THE BOOKS THAT I use for reference in my quest for a longer and happier life are listed below.

Disease Prevention and Treatment, Life Extension Foundation, 1665 pp. This tome came with my membership in Life Extension, and it is a very valuable source of information on diseases and supplements and their uses.

Breakthrough, Eight Steps to Wellness, Life Altering Secrets from Today's Cutting Edge Doctors, Suzanne Somers, 450 pp, Crown Publishers, New York. Highly recommended for anyone interested in cutting edge medicine, or in enjoyably living an extra 10, 20, or 30 years. This is eye-opening for knowledgeable people, and is positively revolutionary for the ordinary person.

The Life Extension Revolution, Philip Lee Miller, MD and the Life Extension Foundation, Bantam Dell, New

York, 2005, 404 pp. This was my first introduction to the idea of extension of life and what it means. A very good book.

The Omega Rx Zone, Dr. Barry Sears, Harper Collins Publishers, 2002, 494 pgs. The major thrust of this book is that high-dose, pharmaceutical grade fish oil can be a major player in the treatment or prevention of many diseases. Dr Sears specifically discusses many diseases that have been helped by his fish oil, like Alzheimer's, other dementias, strokes, ADD and others like it, depression, dyslexia, Parkinson's disease, multiple sclerosis, schizophrenia, and violent behavior.

The Mayo Clinic Plan for Healthy Aging, Edward Creagan, MD, Medical Editor in Chief, Mayo Clinic Health Solutions, 384 pp. To me, this is a valuable source of some information, but I have to keep it in mind that this is the standard medical profession talking through this book. I use it for medical information, but not for dosage.

Discovering the Power Within You, A Guide to the Unexplored Depths Within, Eric Butterworth, a Unity Minister, Harper Collins Publishers, 1992, 239 pgs.

The Secret, Rhonda Byrne, Atria Books/Beyond Words, 2006, 198 pgs.

The Power is Within You, Louise L. Hay, Hay House, Inc., 239 pgs.

Ask and it is Given, Learning to Manifest your Desires, Esther and Jerry Hicks, Hay House, Inc., 314 pgs.

The Language Police, Diane Ravitch, Alfred A. Knopf, 2003, 255 pgs.

I receive multiple emails from Life Extension Foundation on health matters. I print the pertinent ones of these out for my work group, and keep a copy in my own files.

Appendix 1. Vitamin D3

Importance of Vitamin D3

RESEARCH REPORTS KEEP rolling in on the importance of vitamin D3 in our diet, beyond its familiar role in helping us to build strong bones.

Vitamin D3 also helps with: 17 varieties of cancer, heart disease, stroke, hypertension, autoimmune diseases, diabetes, depression, chronic pain, osteoarthritis, osteoporosis, muscle wasting, birth defects, periodontal disease, and apparently helps people live longer.

One strong argument for higher dosage Vitamin D3 is that in equatorial Africa, the birthplace of the human race, the population there now has Vitamin D3 levels in their blood that is in the neighborhood of 50 ng/ml. This is also the level that the present guidelines are recommending. The thinking goes that if natives in Africa have blood levels like that, and they are obviously healthy, then everyone else in the world will benefit from the same levels.

An article in Life Extension Magazine states, "While mainstream doctors are finally realizing the lethal dangers of insufficient Vitamin D3, they still don't understand that optimal levels of Vitamin D3 in the blood are over 50 ng/ml. Achieving this optimal blood level usually requires the daily ingestion of 8,000 IU to 10,000 IU of Vitamin D3. Vitamin D3 has a **MAJOR** benefit to the body, and has been added to my list of supplements that you should be taking.

Recommendations

My recommendations on Vitamin D3 are probably different from anything you have seen or heard before. Recent changes require re-thinking the Vitamin D3 scenario, and adjusting recommendations accordingly.

For example, a few short weeks ago, it was considered appropriate to take Vitamin D3 supplements of 600 IU, or 800 IU for people over 60 (this is the current guidelines of the Food and Nutrition Board). This has now been proven to be woefully inadequate.

Recent changes more than quadruple that, as seen in the Life Extension article. You should be taking about 15,000 IU for a few months, to build up the Vitamin D3 in your blood. Then phase back to about 7,000 to 10,000 IU as a maintenance dose.

As a current example, I was taking about 18,000 IU as a starter base. I am now taking somewhat less as a maintenance dose; 400 IU in my multivitamin, 800 IU in my calcium, and an additional 12,000 IU, for a total of 13,200 IU. Information that I now have indicates that this value is safe. I have recently (2012) been taking about 8500 IU as a maintenance dose; I plan to shortly take a blood test to confirm my blood level is above the minimum.

As an added incentive to you, consider the ability to avoid the flu, colds, and other nasties like them. This level of Vitamin D3 will do it for you. I know; during this past winter, I frequently woke up at night with something like the beginnings of a cold or sore throat, and woke up the next morning with no sign of anything out of the ordinary. And I recently had several occurrences of coughing during the night; a weird cough not like anything I ever had before. But it was completely gone the next morning. And as an added inducement, I recently (2011) had a blood test that revealed my current blood level of Vitamin D3; it was 67ng/ml, safely above the recommended minimum.

If you follow my recommendations, then you should not have to take further precautions. However, if you find it convenient, or you want personal reassurance, then you should get a blood test done. If so, I would highly recommend Life Extension Foundation; they offer an inexpensive blood test. And if you still need reassurance, talk to your regular doctor or other health provider. If you don't like what he/she is telling you, you can always find yourself another doctor.

So turn on to Vitamin D3 and enjoy a lot more in life.

Appendix 2. Vitamin K

ANOTHER SHOE JUST dropped; you need Vitamin K in addition to Vitamin D3. It turns out that Vitamin K is a helper to Vitamin D3; Vitamin K plays a critical role in maintaining healthy bone density by facilitating the transport of calcium from the bloodstream into the bones. Vitamin K is also required by calcium-regulating proteins in the arteries. So Vitamin K has been added to my list of **MAJOR** supplements that you should be taking.

Vitamin K comes in 3 flavors, K1, MK-4, and MK-7, and all 3 flavors are valuable in the body. However, only K1 is available from normal diet sources, but very little of that is actually absorbed in the body; K1 is usually bound too tight to the vegetable molecules.

The main source of Vitamin K that I know of and would presently recommend is from Life Extension (http://www.lef.org/ or dial 1-800-544-4440 for Super K with Advanced K2 Complex. This has all 3 flavors of

Vitamin K in it, in about the same ratio needed by the body.

In the case of Vitamin K, please note that still another shoe is in the process of dropping. According to an article in the November 2010 copy of Life Extension Magazine, Vitamin K is an excellent cancer fighter. It both prevents and treats many kinds of cancer. The summary in the article is revealing:

Cancer remains a deadly threat for millions of aging Americans, despite decades of aggressive research. Standard cancer medications can only help after a cancer is discovered, and even then they are limited by toxicity. Standard cancer treatments attack only one or a few biochemical steps in the long cascade of events leading to tumor development.

Long associated only with blood clotting, vitamin K is now known to have effects on tissues throughout the body, including most of the steps leading up to cancer. Recent discoveries about Vitamin K illustrate the tremendous breadth of its targets, spanning virtually every phase in cancer's deadly progress. A solid base of laboratory science is complemented by compelling clinical evidence that Vitamin K can prevent, and in some cases treat, a variety of common and dangerous cancers.

Need I say more? If you have any doubts about this, please call the Life Extension Health Advisor at 1-866-864-3027. If they ask you for an ID, then just tell them you are an associate of mine.

Appendix 3. Metformin

ANOTHER SHOE IS now in the process of dropping; you might need to add the diabetes drug Metformin to your pill box. According to an article in the November 2010 copy of Life Extension Magazine, Metformin is an excellent cancer fighter.

Metformin is like Vitamin K in its actions on cancer. It currently fights Breast Cancer, Endometrial Cancer, Prostate Cancer, Pancreatic Cancer, and Colon Cancer. It probably fights almost every developmental stage in almost every cancer in existence. This is currently being tested in many laboratories in the world, so stay tuned on this one.

Metformin is a prescription drug, currently the most popular diabetes drug, taken by thousands if not millions of people. The generic version of this is available and currently inexpensive, so a prescription from your doctor for this should not break the bank.

You should take Metformin even if you are not currently a diabetic. Along with Vitamin K, Metformin is extremely valuable as a cancer fighter and preventer. Its effects are currently **MAJOR**, and will probably get better as new experiments get reported. Metformin has been added to my list of supplements that you should be taking.

Appendix 4. Aspirin

THINK YOU KNEW everything about Aspirin? I did, but I am still finding out things that surprise me. For example, I knew it was a "drug" that you should be taking every day, but I did not know the details of just why that was true.

An article in Life Extension Magazine, May 2011, gave me the added details, and these are details that you should also know and act on. The detail summary is as follows:

- *Aspirin can reduce your overall risk of death by all forms of cancer by 20%.*

- *Aspirin can reduce your risk of colorectal cancer death by up to 40%.*

- *To achieve these protective effects, only a "baby aspirin" containing 75 mg to 81 mg needs to be taken every day. Or, if you are like me and already had a stroke, take a standard 325 mg Aspirin each day.*

- *To achieve these protective effects, take the Aspirin for the rest of your life. The cancer protective effects noted above begin after you have been on Aspirin for about 5 years, and increase from there to their maximum effect at about 10 years of use. Which is good news to me, since I have been on Aspirin for about 12 years.*

- *This protective effect increased with age, and was especially effective in those 55 years old and older.*

- *The protective effects of Aspirin will continue as long as you keep taking it.*

For some of you, this news will be welcome and be easily incorporated into your daily life. For others, there may be complications of taking Aspirin. It might cause stomach distress or even ulcers, might cause kidney problems, or might cause other system upsets or outright disasters. So heed my advice and talk to your doctor before going on any Aspirin regimen. If you need arguments to support your desire, then show him or her this copy and quote the Life Extension article mentioned above. He or she should be able to find this article in the local library.

If you have problems taking Aspirin, you can reduce the effects of taking Aspirin by: 1) taking the smallest dose that you can, the 75 mg or 81 mg dose, the so-called baby Aspirin; 2) take the anti-ulcer supplement Zinc Carnosine (polaprezinc); or 3) take cranberries or licorice extracts to prevent H. Pylori, the bug that often causes stomach ulcers.

Appendix 5. Resveratrol

IN 1997, THE first study of the effects of Resveratrol was published. Since then, there has been an intense study of the medical effects of Resveratrol. There was a Resveratrol Conference held in 2010, and the conference results were published in 2011. The primary objective of this conference was to examine the totality of the evidence for any disease-preventing role of resveratrol in aging humans. About 3650 published studies were analyzed and reported on.

This paper is a summary of an article in Life Extension magazine, March 2012, in which the conference results were reported. If you want more details than is given here, please see the original article. If you can find no other source, the magazine should be available in your local library, or call Life Extension at 1-800-544-4440.

As you will discover in this summary, the medical role of Resveratrol is now proven to be **MAJOR**. There are 12 mechanisms of action by which Resveratrol acts to combat the killer diseases of aging and to delay the aging process itself. You will also discover data on the 5 leading causes of death among Americans, including heart disease, cancer, neurodegenaration, systemic inflammation, obesity, and diabetes.

For the 12 key anti-aging mechanisms of Resveratrol, please see Table 1. For the protective effects of resveratrol in 5 leading causes of death, please see Table 2.

TABLE 1. RESVERATROL'S 12 KEY MECHANISMS

MECHANISM	DISEASES OR CONDITIONS AFFECTED
•Modulation of oxidation/ antioxidation status	All chronic diseases
•Suppression of inflammation	All chronic diseases
•Mitochodndrial protection •Suppression of fat cell formation and stimulation of fat breakdown	Obesity, diabetes, cardiovascular disease
•Modulation of cell proliferation and apoptosis (programmed cell death) •Inhibition of metastasis •Modulation of DNA damage •Modulation of foreign molecule and toxin metabolism	Cancer
•Modulation of glutamate (excitatory neurotransmitter) mechanism	Neurodegenerative diseases
•Estrogenic activity/ anti-estrogenic activity	Multiple hormone dependent cancers
•Stimulation of bone formation	Bone health and osteoporosis

TABLE 2. RESVERATROL'S EFFECTS IN LEADING CAUSES OF DEATH

CONDITION	MECHANISM
Heart Disease	Reduces incidence of hypertension, heart failure, ischemia (loss of blood flow)
Cancer	Chemoprevention
Stroke	Reduces incidence of hypertension, ischemia, is neuroprotective
Neurodegenerative diseases (e.g. Alzheimer's, Parkinson's), brain injury	Neuroprotective
Diabetes (and obesity)	Improves insulin sensitivity, reduces blood glucose levels, reduces high-fat diet-induced obesity and visceral (abdominal) fat

Appendix 6. Glutathione

THE FOLLOWING MATERIAL has been extracted from another good book, The Immortality Edge by Greta Blackburn, Michael Fossel, and Dave Woynorowski. Greta Blackburn is the principal author, and it is she that won the Nobel Prize for Chemistry for defining that telomeres define aging.

According to this book, Glutathione is a master molecule in the body, necessary for many body functions. It is extremely hard to supplement, though. Taking it by mouth by capsules or pills of any kind does not work; acids in the stomach and intestines destroy it. Injections of glutathione also do not work very well; enzymes in the blood also destroy most of it.

Glutathione does many things for your body, most of them important. Glutathione detoxifies the body and helps it repair damage caused by stress, pollution radiation, infection, drugs, poor diet, aging, injury, trauma, and burns. Glutathione improves heart function, improves blood sugar numbers in diabetes, and improves response to exercise. Glutathione also aids in a process called autophagy, which recycles dead and dying cells to manufacture new cells. Glutathione also helps keep the mitochondria in each of your cells healthy and producing as they should.

I am aware of only 2 methods of supplementing Glutathione, and you should take one of them to be certain that your own levels of Glutathione are sufficient for your health. 1) Take N-Acetylcysteine (NAC), which is rapidly metabolized in the body, where it becomes a precursor to intercellular Glutathione. NAC is available locally from Vitamin World in Rockvale Square, or from http://www.vitaminworld.com/. 2) A cream containing Dipalmitoyl Glutathione and called Protect 120 is now available from a special source, Stem Cell Products, 3350 Palm Center Drive, Las Vegas NV, http://www.stem120,com/. You simply rub about an inch of this cream on your arm each day.

Please note that I am now taking both approaches to an adequate supply of Glutathione. Needless to say, I plan to be around and still be enjoying life for the next 20 (or more) years.

Please note also that Glutathione is not available in a pill of any kind; you should NOT buy such pills, since they are worthless. I recently saw a bottle of pills like this in Wal-Mart, and guess what I did not buy. My strong recommendation to you is to buy bottles of NAC and let nature take its course; let nature provide the Glutathione that you very much need.